INTRODUCTION TO THE
PSYCHOLOGY OF LEARNING

INTRODUCTION TO THE PSYCHOLOGY OF HEARING

BRIAN C. J. MOORE, M.A., Ph.D.

Lecturer, Department of Psychology,
University of Cambridge

UNIVERSITY PARK PRESS

BALTIMORE · LONDON · TOKYO

First published 1977 by
The Macmillan Press Ltd
London and Basingstoke

Published in North America by
UNIVERSITY PARK PRESS
Chamber of Commerce Building
Baltimore, Maryland 21202

Printed in Great Britain

Library of Congress Cataloging in Publication Data

Moore, Brian C   J
    Introduction to the psychology of hearing.

    Bibliography: p.
    Includes index.
    1. Auditory perception. 2. Hearing.
I. Title. [DNLM: 1. Hearing. 2. Psycho-
acoustics. WV270 M821i]
BF251.M66 1977   152.1'5   76–30756
ISBN 0-8391-0996-2

To Carol

Contents

7

Contents

Preface

In 1971 I gave my first course of lectures on auditory perception, as part of the psychology course at the University of Reading. Anyone who has attempted to give or attend lectures on auditory perception will be aware of two major problems which I encountered. Firstly, there is no textbook which is both up to date and at a level suitable for undergraduate use. Secondly, scientific papers on hearing in psychological and physiological journals are almost incomprehensible to the beginner in this area. I became increasingly frustrated at having to say to my students 'I'm sorry, but there is no book I can recommend,' and finally I decided that the only solution to the problem was to write such a book myself.

This book, then, is primarily intended as an undergraduate textbook to accompany courses in auditory perception or hearing. To this end it contains a chapter introducing the basic physics of sound and describing the most important anatomical and physiological features of the auditory system. Some very basic knowledge is assumed (for example, the terms 'neurone' and 'nerve firings' are not explained), but the approach is very much to start from first principles.

As it turned out, the book contains very much more material than I would normally get through in a single course of lectures, so that it could also serve as a text to accompany advanced undergraduate or graduate courses in auditory perception. The general approach throughout the book is to relate the psychological and perceptual aspects of sound to the underlying physiological mechanisms. Thus the book should also be of use and interest to sensory physiologists, physicians and audiologists.

Although the emphasis throughout the book is on laboratory experiments performed under carefully controlled conditions, I have

11

been careful to point out, wherever possible, the real-life or applied relevance of the problems under discussion. Indeed the final chapter of the book is mainly concerned with practical applications. In addition, there is a chapter on speech perception in which links with psychoacoustic phenomena are emphasised. Thus the book should also have something of interest for phoneticians, speech researchers, speech pathologists, linguists, and engineers concerned with problems of the recording, transmission and reproduction of sound or with problems of automatic speech recognition and speaker identification.

My major aim in writing this book was that it should be reasonably up to date, but at the same time not too technical for the novice. Inevitably this has resulted in the omission of some details and the simplification of some concepts. I hope that I have managed to do this without too much distortion, and that the essential flavour of current trends in auditory research has been preserved. Many areas which are traditionally discussed in textbooks on hearing have been omitted entirely; for example, volume and density as attributes of pure tones are not mentioned, nor is the mel scale of pitch. This reflects my own prejudices to some extent, but the basis for omission has generally been the lack of use of these concepts in the last ten years or so.

Perhaps the hardest thing about writing this book was to stop writing it! Almost every day I came across new papers with exciting results which ought to have been mentioned. However, one has to draw the line somewhere, and the book was never intended to be a complete review. I apologise to those whose work has been omitted or mentioned too briefly. The balance of space has inevitably been influenced by my own interests, and I hope that I will be forgiven for devoting so much space to the role of 'timing' information in nerve impulses.

Auditory perception has been a sadly neglected area in British psychology, although this is much less true in the United States and Holland. I hope that this book will help to correct the balance, and that those who teach in this area will find the book of some use.

Finally, I would like to thank all those colleagues and friends who read parts of the manuscript and provided helpful comments. The manuscript was written while I was a lecturer in Psychology at the University of Reading. Thanks are due particularly to: Mark Haggard, Max Coltheart, Bernard Moulden, Alan Allport, David

Raab, Roy Davis, Wynford Bellin, Mark Terry, Peter Bailey, Arthur Summerfield, Dave Martin, John Gundry, Carol Moore and Pat Sheldon. The responsibility for mistakes is of course mine. Mrs P. Williams typed the manuscript accurately and quickly through many drafts to its final form; I am very grateful to her. Susan and Paul Scott, and my wife, Carol, provided valuable help in sorting out the references.

Reading, 1977   B. C. J. M.

1

The Nature of Sound and the Structure of the Auditory System

1.1. INTRODUCTION

One of the general aims of this book is to specify, as far as possible, the relationships between the characteristics of the sounds which enter the ear and the sensations which they produce. Wherever possible these relationships will be specified in terms of the underlying mechanisms. In other words, we will be trying to understand how the auditory system works, as well as to look at what it does. It is not always possible to fulfil both of these objectives. While some aspects of auditory perception can be explained by reference to the anatomy or physiology of the auditory system, our knowledge in this respect is not usually as precise or as far reaching as we would like. Often the results of behavioural studies (generally psychophysical experiments) provide us with evidence as to the kinds of things which are occurring in the auditory system, but we may not be able to specify the detailed physiological mechanisms which are involved. Sometimes we can use the results of psychophysical experiments to determine whether a particular type of neural coding (see later), which in principle could convey information about a sound, is actually involved in the perception or discrimination of that sound. Before we can begin to specify underlying mechanisms, however, we must know something of the physical nature of sounds, and of the basic anatomy and physiology of the auditory system. That is the purpose of this chapter.

1.2 THE PHYSICAL CHARACTERISTICS OF SOUNDS

Sound originates from the motion or vibration of an object. This motion is impressed upon the surrounding medium (usually air) in

15

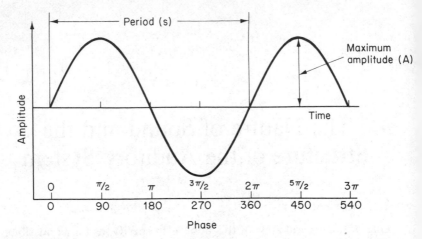

Figure 1.1 The waveform of a sine wave or sinusoidal vibration. Only $1\frac{1}{2}$ cycles are shown, although the waveform should be pictured as repeating indefinitely. The instantaneous amplitude is given by the expression $A \sin (2\pi ft)$, where t = time, f = frequency and A = maximum amplitude. Phase is indicated along the bottom, using as a reference point the first zero-crossing of the wave. Phase may be measured in degrees or in radians. One complete cycle corresponds to 360 degrees or 2π radians.

the form of alternate waves of compression and rarefaction. What actually happens is that the atmospheric particles, or molecules, are squeezed closer together than normal, and then pulled farther apart than normal. Thus a sound wave moves outwards from the vibrating body, but the molecules do not advance with the wave: they vibrate about an average resting place. The sound wave generally weakens as it moves away from the source, and also may be subject to reflections and refractions caused by walls or objects in its path. Thus the sound 'image' reaching the ear will differ somewhat from that initially generated.

One of the simplest type of sound is the sine wave, also known as a sinusoidal vibration, which has the waveform (pressure variation plotted against time) shown in Figure 1.1. This wave is simple both from the physical and mathematical point of view and from the point of view of the auditory system. It happens that sine waves produce particularly simple responses in the auditory system, and that they have a very 'clean' or 'pure' sound, like that of a tuning fork. Thus they are also called simple tones or pure tones. To describe a sine wave we need to specify three things: the *frequency*, or the number of times per second the waveform repeats itself (specified in cycles per second, or Hertz, where 1 Hertz (Hz) equals 1 c/s); the *amplitude*, or the amount of pressure variation about the mean or normal; the *phase*, or the portion of the cycle through which the wave has advanced in relation to some fixed point in time. For continuous sinusoids phase is only a relevant parameter when we are interested in the relationship between two or more different waves. The time taken for one complete cycle of the waveform is called the period, which is the reciprocal of the frequency.

A sine wave is not the only kind of sound which repeats regularly. Many of the sounds which we encounter in everyday life, such as those produced by musical instruments, and certain speech sounds, also show such regularity, and hence are called periodic sounds. Although these sounds are generally more complex than sine waves, they share a common subjective characteristic with sine waves in that they have pitches. Pitch may be defined as that attribute of auditory sensation in terms of which sounds may be ordered on a musical scale. In other words, pitch is that attribute the variation of which constitutes melody. Any sound which produces a pitch may be called a tone. In general, tones are periodic, but as we shall see later, this is not always the case.

The pitch of a sound is related to its repetition rate and, hence, in the case of a sine wave, to frequency. It should be emphasised that pitch is a subjective property of a stimulus, and as such cannot be measured directly. However, for a sine wave the pitch is closely related to the frequency; the higher the frequency, the higher the pitch. For a more complex sound the pitch is often investigated by asking the subject to adjust a sine wave so that it has the same pitch as the complex sound. The frequency of the sine wave is then taken as a measure of the pitch of the complex sound.

Although all sounds can be specified in terms of variations in sound pressure occurring over time, it is often more convenient, and more meaningful, to specify them in a different way when the sounds are complex. This method is based on a theorem by Fourier, who proved that any complex waveform (with certain restrictions) can be analysed, or broken down, into a series of sine waves with specific frequencies, amplitudes and phases. Such an analysis is called Fourier analysis, and each sine wave is called a frequency (or Fourier) component of the complex sound. The frequency components are also sometimes called partials. We may thus define a complex tone as a tone composed of a number of simple tones, or sine waves.

The simplest type of complex tone to which Fourier analysis can be applied is one which is *periodic*. Such a tone is composed of a number of simple tones each of which has a frequency which is an exact multiple of some common (not necessarily present) fundamental component. The fundamental component thus has the lowest frequency of any of the components in the complex tone, and it may be said to form the 'foundation' for the other components. The fundamental component has a frequency equal to the repetition rate of the complex waveform as a whole. The frequency components, or partials, of the complex tone are known as harmonics, and are numbered, the fundamental being given harmonic number 1. Thus, for example, a note of middle C played on the piano would have a fundamental component or first harmonic of frequency 256 Hz, a second harmonic of frequency 512 Hz, a third harmonic of frequency 768 Hz, etc. The nth harmonic has a frequency which is n times that of the fundamental. An illustration of how a complex tone can be built up from a series of sine waves is given in Figure 1.2.

One of the reasons for representing sounds in this way is that humans do seem to be able to hear the harmonics of a periodic sound wave individually to a limited extent. For example, Mersenne (1636) stated that 'the string struck and sounded freely makes at least five sounds at the same time, the first of which is the natural sound of the string and serves as the foundation for the rest . . .' The phenomenon that humans can hear out the sinusoidal components of a complex tone is known as Ohm's Acoustical Law, after the German physicist Georg Ohm. Normally, when we are presented with a complex tone, we do not listen in this way, but nevertheless we do appear to be *able* to hear out the lower harmonics of a complex sound to some extent (see Chapters 3 and 4 for further discussion of this). When we are presented with two simultaneous pure tones, whose frequencies are not too similar, then these will often be heard as two separate sounds rather than as a single complex sound. Thus our perception corresponds to the analysis of the sound in terms of its Fourier components. Notice that our perception of colour is quite different; if lights of two different frequencies (or wavelengths) are mixed, we see a single colour corresponding to the mixture, rather than seeing two component hues.

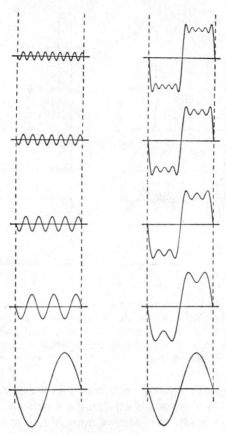

Figure 1.2 An illustration of how a complex waveform (a square wave) can be built up from a series of sinusoidal components. The square wave is composed of odd harmonics only, and the 1st, 3rd, 5th, 7th and 9th harmonics are shown on the left. The series on the right shows progressive changes from a simple sine wave as each component is added. If enough additional harmonics, with appropriate amplitudes and phases, were added, the composite wave would approach a perfectly square shape. From Newman (1948), by permission of John Wiley & Sons (Inc.), New York.

The structure of a sound, in terms of its frequency component, is often represented by its frequency spectrum—a plot of sound amplitude (or energy) against frequency. Examples of frequency spectra are given in Figure 1.3. For periodic sounds of long duration, the

19

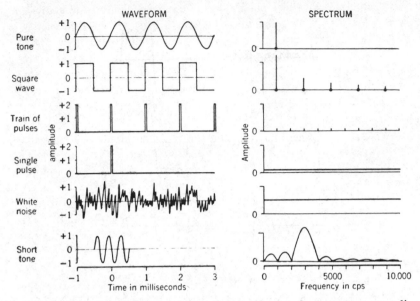

Figure 1.3 On the left are shown the waveforms of some common auditory stimuli, and on the right are the corresponding spectra. The periodic stimuli (pure tone, square wave and train of pulses) have line spectra, while the non-periodic stimuli (single pulse, white noise and short tone burst) have continuous spectra.

energy falls at specific discrete frequencies and the spectrum is known as a line spectrum. For sounds which are not periodic, such as white noise (a hissing sound), or sounds of finite duration, such as a click or a short burst of a tone, the spectrum tends to be more complex, and is obtained by use of a mathematical device known as the Fourier Transform. Spectra of such sounds are known as continuous spectra; the energy is spread over certain frequency bands, rather than being concentrated at particular frequencies. Some examples of this type are also given in Figure 1.3. Notice that a short burst of a sinusoid (often called a tone pulse) has a frequency spectrum containing energy over a wide range of frequencies. Although the peak in the spectrum occurs at the nominal frequency of the tone pulse, there is considerable energy at other frequencies. This spread of energy increases as the duration of the tone pulse is shortened. Corresponding changes occur in our perception of such tone pulses; as a tone pulse is shortened in duration, it becomes less tone-like and more click-like.

20

In general, whenever a stimulus is changed abruptly (e.g. by a change in level or a change in frequency), a spread in spectral energy occurs. This spreading of spectral energy over frequency is often called 'energy splatter'. Energy splatter can be reduced, by slowing down the changes (e.g. by switching tones on and off gradually), but it cannot be completely eliminated. We shall see later that energy splatter may play an important role in studies of masking and of pitch discrimination.

In many psychoacoustic experiments the experimenter may desire to manipulate the spectra of the stimuli in some way. For example, he may wish to remove certain frequency components from a complex stimulus while leaving other components unchanged. In practice this is usually achieved by altering the electrical signal before it is converted into sound by a loudspeaker or headphone. The electronic devices which may be used to manipulate the spectrum of a signal are known as filters. A high-pass filter removes all frequency components below a certain cut-off frequency, but does not affect components above this frequency. A low-pass filter does the reverse. A band-pass filter has two cut-off frequencies, passing components between these two frequencies and removing components outside this range. A band-stop filter also has two cut-off frequencies, but it removes components between these two frequencies, leaving other components intact. In practice it is not possible to design filters with a perfectly sharp cut-off; instead there will be a range of frequencies over which some frequency components are reduced in level but not entirely removed. Thus, in order to specify a filter, we have to state not only the cut-off frequency (or frequencies) but also the sharpness of the cut-off or the 'slope' of the filter. Some typical filter characteristics are illustrated in Figure 1.4. Notice that if a signal with a 'flat' spectrum, such as white noise, is passed through a filter, the spectrum of the output of the filter will have the same shape (i.e. be the same function of frequency) as the filter characteristic. Thus we can also talk of a high-pass noise, a band-pass noise, etc. Any alteration of the spectrum of a signal by filtering also produces a corresponding alteration in the waveform of the signal, and usually an alteration in the way it is perceived. For example, if white noise is band-pass filtered, it assumes a pitch-like quality, the pitch corresponding to the centre frequency of the filter.

Let us now turn to the measurement of sound levels. The instruments used to measure these, such as microphones, normally respond

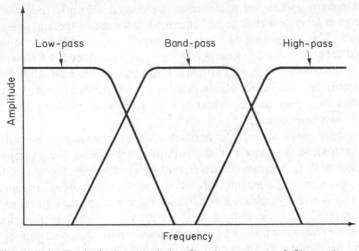

Figure 1.4 Typical characteristics for three types of filters: low-pass, band-pass and high-pass. The input to each filter is a sinusoid of constant amplitude but variable frequency. The amplitude of the output of each filter is plotted as a function of frequency.

to changes in air pressure, and thus give an output proportional to the amplitude of the sound. We use the term 'amplitude' here to refer to deviations in pressure from the mean value (normal atmospheric pressure). However, it is more usual to specify sound levels in terms of intensity, which is the sound power transmitted through a given area in a sound field. For a medium such as air there is a simple relationship between the amplitude of a plane (flat-fronted) sound wave in a free field (i.e. in the absence of reflected sound) and the acoustic intensity; intensity is proportional to the square of amplitude.

It turns out that the auditory system can deal with a huge range of sound intensities (see Chapter 2). This makes it inconvenient to deal with sound intensities or powers directly. Instead a logarithmic scale expressing the *ratio* of two intensities is used. One intensity is chosen as a reference level, I_0, and the other intensity, I_1, is expressed relative to this. One Bel corresponds to a ratio of intensities of 10:1. Thus the number of Bels corresponding to a given intensity ratio is obtained by taking the logarithm to the base 10 of the intensity ratio. For example, an intensity ratio of 100:1 corresponds to 2 Bels. Unfortunately, the Bel is a rather large unit for everyday use, and to

22

obtain units of convenient size the Bel is divided into 10 decibels (dB). Thus the number of decibels corresponding to a given ratio of acoustic intensity is

$$\text{number of dB} = 10 \log_{10} (I_1/I_0).$$

Notice that a given number of dB represents an intensity or power ratio, not an absolute intensity. In order to specify the absolute intensity of a sound it is necessary to state that the intensity (or power) of the sound, I_1, is N dB above or below some reference level I_0. The reference level most commonly used is an intensity of 10^{-16} watts per square centimetre (W/cm²), which is equivalent to a pressure of 0.0002 dynes per square centimetre (dyn/cm²). The reference sound pressure is now commonly expressed in the International System of Units (SI) as 2×10^{-5} N/m² or 20 μPa (micropascal). A sound level specified using this reference level is referred to as a Sound Pressure Level (SPL). Thus a sound at 60 dB SPL is 60 dB higher in level than the reference level of 0 dB (10^{-16} W/cm²), and has an intensity of 10^{-10} W/cm². Notice that multiplying (or dividing) the ratio of intensities by 10 increases (or decreases) the number of dB by 10. It is also convenient to remember that a twofold change in intensity corresponds to a change in level of 3 dB.

The reference sound level, 0 dB SPL, is a low sound level which was chosen to be close to the average human absolute threshold for a 1000 Hz pure tone. The absolute threshold is the minimum detectable level of a sound in the absence of any other external sounds (the manner of presentation of the sound and method of determining detectability must be specified). In fact the average human absolute threshold at 1000 Hz is about 6.5 dB SPL. Sometimes it is convenient to choose as a reference level the threshold of a subject for the sound being used. A sound level specified in this way is referred to as a Sensation Level (SL). Thus, for a given subject, a sound at 60 dB SL will be 60 dB above the absolute threshold of that subject for that sound. The physical intensity corresponding to a given Sensation Level will, of course, differ from subject to subject, and from sound to sound.

Finally, it is useful to adapt the decibel notation so that it expresses ratios of pressure as well as ratios of intensity. This may be done by recalling that intensity is proportional to the square of pressure. If one sound has an intensity of I_1 and an amplitude (pressure) A_1,

Table 1.1   The relationship between decibels, intensity ratios and amplitude ratios. Sound levels in dB SPL are expressed relatively to a level I_0 of of 10^{-16} W/cm^2. This is equivalent to 2×10^{-5} N/m^2, or 0.0002 dyn/cm^2. 10^n means 1 followed by n zeros

Sound level, dB SPL	Intensity ratio, I/I_0	Amplitude ratio, A/A_0	Typical example
180	10^{18}	10^9	Saturn rocket from 150 ft
140	10^{14}	10^7	Loud rock group
100	10^{10}	10^5	Shouting at close range
80	10^8	10^4	Busy street
70	10^7	3.2×10^3	Normal conversation
50	10^5	316	Quiet conversation
30	10^3	31.6	Soft whisper
20	100	10	Country area at night
6.5	4.5	2.1	Mean threshold at 1 kHz
3	2	1.4	
0	1	1	Reference level I_0
-10	0.1	0.32	
-60	10^{-6}	10^{-3}	

and a second sound has an intensity I_2 and amplitude A_2, then the difference in level between them is

$$\text{number of dB} = 10 \log_{10}(I_1/I_2) = 10 \log_{10}(A_1/A_2)^2$$
$$= 20 \log_{10}(A_1/A_2).$$

Thus a tenfold increase in amplitude (pressure) corresponds to a hundredfold increase in intensity and is represented by $+20$ dB. Table 1.1 gives some examples of intensity and pressure ratios expressed in decibels, and also indicates sound levels, in dB SPL, corresponding to various common sounds.

Finally, under the physics of sound, it is useful to define what is meant by a *linear* system. For a system to be linear two conditions must be satisfied. Firstly, the output of the system in response to a

24

number of independent inputs presented simultaneously should be equal to the sum of the outputs that would have been obtained if each input were presented alone. Secondly, if the input to the system is changed in magnitude by a factor k, then the output should also change in magnitude by a factor k, but be otherwise unaltered. These two conditions are known as superposition and homogeneity, respectively. In a linear system, if the input is doubled, then the ontput is doubled, but without any change in the form of the output. Further, the output of a linear system *never* contains frequency components that were not present in the input signal. Thus a sinusoidal input gives rise to a sinusoidal output. This is not necessarily true for other types of waveforms. We shall see later that some parts of the auditory system behave as though they were approximately linear, while others behave in a grossly non-linear way.

1.3 BASIC STRUCTURE OF THE AUDITORY SYSTEM

Figure 1.5 shows the structure of the peripheral part of the human auditory system. The outer ear is composed of the pinna (the part we actually see) and the auditory canal or meatus. The pinna has generally been considered a rather unimportant part of the auditory system, but it does in fact significantly modify the incoming sound, particularly at high frequencies, and this is important in our ability to localise sounds (see Chapter 5). Sound travels down the meatus and causes the eardrum, or tympanic membrane, to vibrate. These vibrations are transmitted through the middle ear by three small bones, the ossicles, to a membrane-covered opening in the bony wall of the spiral-shaped structure of the inner ear—cochlea. This opening is called the oval window. The three bones are called the malleus, incus and stapes, the stapes being the lightest and smallest of these, and the one which actually makes contact with the oval window. The major function of the middle ear is to ensure the efficiency transfer of sound from the air to the fluids in the cochlea. If the sound were to impinge directly onto the oval window, most of it would simply be reflected back, rather than entering the cochlea. The middle ear acts as an impedance-matching device or transformer to improve sound transmission. This is accomplished mainly by the difference in effective areas of the eardrum and the oval window, and to a small extent by the lever action of the ossicles.

The ossicles have minute muscles attached to them which contract

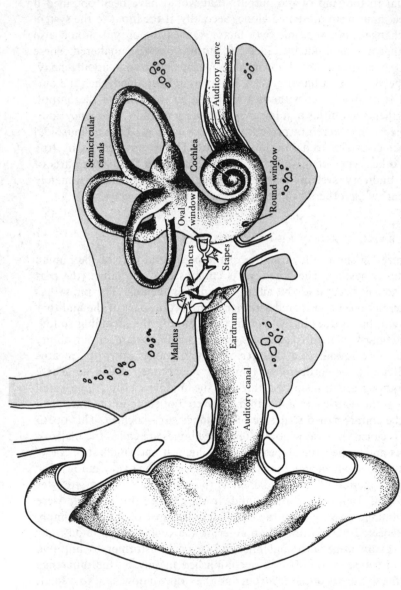

Figure 1.5 Illustration of the structure of the peripheral auditory system showing the outer, middle and inner ear. From *Human Information Processing*, by Lindsey, P. H. and Norman, D. A. (1972), by permission of the authors and Academic Press.

Labels in figure: Semicircular canals, Cochlea, Auditory nerve, Round window, Oval window, Stapes, Incus, Malleus, Eardrum, Auditory canal when we are exposed to intense sounds. This contraction, known as the middle-ear reflex, is probably mediated by neural centres in the brain-stem, but its anatomical basis is not fully known. The reflex reduces the transmission of sound through the middle ear, particularly at low frequencies, and it may help to prevent damage to the delicate structures of the cochlea.

The cochlea is the most important part of the ear from our point of view, and an understanding of what goes on in the cochlea can provide a key to many aspects of auditory perception. The cochlea is filled with incompressible fluids, and it also has bony rigid walls. It is divided along its length by two membranes, Reissner's membrane and the basilar membrane (see Figure 1.11). It is the motion of the basilar membrane in response to sound which is of primary interest to us. The start of the cochlea, where the oval window is situated, is known as the base, while the other end, the inner tip, is known as the apex. At the apex there is a small opening (the helicotrema) between the basilar membrane and the walls of the cochlea, so that fluid can flow between the two main chambers of the cochlea, the scala vestibuli and the scala tympani. Inward movement of the oval window results in a flow of fluid around the helicotrema and a corresponding outward movement in a membrane covering a second opening in the cochlea—the round window.

When the oval window is set in motion by an incoming sound, a pressure is applied by the fluids in the cochlea essentially simultaneously along the whole length of the basilar membrane. The pattern of motion on the basilar membrane, however, takes some time to develop. The pattern which occurs does not depend on which end of the cochlea is stimulated. Sounds which reach the cochlea via the bones of the head rather than through the air (e.g. our own voices) do not produce atypical responses.

The response of the basilar membrane to sinusoidal stimulation begins as a bulge at the basal end. This bulge takes the form of a travelling wave which moves along the basilar membrane towards the apex. The amplitude of the wave increases slowly at first and then decreases rather abruptly. This is illustrated in Figure 1.6, which shows the instantaneous displacement of the basilar membrane (derived from a cochlear model) for two successive instants in time. This figure also shows the line joining the amplitude peaks, which is called the envelope. The distance between peaks or zero-crossings in the wave decreases as the wave travels along,

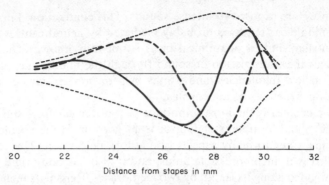

Distance from stapes in mm

Figure 1.6 The instantaneous displacement of the cochlear partition at two successive instants in time, derived from a cochlear model. The pattern moves from left to right, building up gradually with distance, and decaying rapidly beyond the point of maximal displacement. The dotted line represents the envelope traced out by the amplitude peaks in the waveform. From von Békésy (1947), by permission of the *Journal of the Acoustical Society of America*.

and the envelope shows a peak at a particular position on the basilar membrane.

The response of the basilar membrane to sounds of different frequencies is strongly affected by its mechanical properties, which vary considerably from base to apex. At the base it is relatively narrow and stiff, while at the apex it is wider and much less stiff. The position of the peak in the pattern of vibration thus differs according to the frequency of stimulation. High-frequency sounds produce a maximum displacement of the basilar membrane near the oval window, so that there is little activity on the remainder of the membrane. Low-frequency sounds produce a pattern of vibration which extends all the way along the basilar membrane, but which reaches a maximum before the end of the membrane. Figure 1.7 shows the envelopes of the patterns of vibration for several different low-frequency sinusoids (from von Békésy, 1960). It is clear that sounds of different frequencies produce maximum activity at different places along the basilar membrane. In effect the ear is behaving like a Fourier analyser, although with a much less than perfect frequency-analysing power.

It is worth noting that in response to steady sinusoidal stimulation each point on the basilar membrane vibrates in a sinusoidal manner with a frequency equal to that of the input waveform. For example, if we apply a 1000 Hz pure tone, each point on the basilar membrane

28

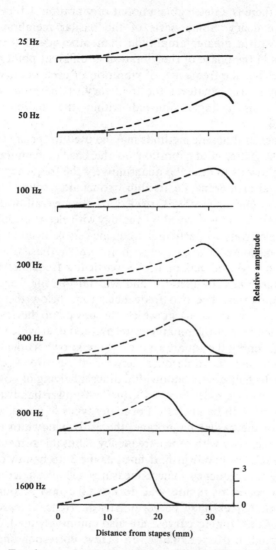

Figure 1.7 Envelopes of patterns of vibration on the basilar membrane for a number of low-frequency sounds. Solid lines indicate the results of actual measurements, while the dashed lines are von Békésy's extrapolations. From *Experiments in Hearing* by von Békésy, G. (1960), used with the permission of McGraw-Hill Book Co.

for which there is a detectable amount of vibration will be vibrating at that frequency. Some parts of the basilar membrane will be vibrating with a greater amplitude than others, and there will be differences in the phase of the vibration at different points along the membrane, but the frequency of vibration of each point will be the same. This is true whatever the frequency of the input waveform, provided it is a single sinusoid within the audible range of frequencies.

A number of different methods may be used to specify the 'sharpness' of the patterns of vibration on the basilar membrane. These methods allow us to describe quantitatively the frequency resolution of the basilar membrane, i.e. its ability to separate sounds of differing frequencies. One measure is related to the overall width of the 'tuning curve', and is derived by analogy with electronic filters which respond selectively to particular frequencies (see Section 1.2). Consider the response at a particular point on the basilar membrane. The response will be maximal for a particular frequency (which we will call the centre frequency), and will fall off for frequencies on either side of this. The two frequencies (one below the centre frequency and one above it) at which the power of the response has fallen to one-half of the maximum response (i.e. at which the amplitude has fallen by the square root of 2) are known as the half-power frequencies, and the difference between these two frequencies is known as the half-power bandwidth. Since a halving of power corresponds to a change in level of 3 dB, the half-power bandwidth is also known as the 3 dB bandwidth. For many types of filters, and for the response of the basilar membrane, the 3 dB bandwidth is not constant, but increases with centre frequency. Thus it is sometimes useful to use the relative bandwidth, defined as the 3 dB bandwidth divided by the centre frequency. These measures tell us something of the overall sharpness of tuning, but do not take into account the fact that 'tuning curves' may be asymmetrical. Hence, measures of the 'slopes' of the 'tuning curves' are also commonly used. The slopes are measured in dB per octave, an octave corresponding to a frequency ratio of 2:1. A slope of 10 dB/octave would mean that the power increased (or decreased) by a factor of 10 for each doubling (or halving) of frequency.

Most of the pioneering work on patterns of vibration along the basilar membrane was done by von Békésy (1928, 1942). His technique involved the use of a light microscope and stroboscopic illumination, to measure the vibration amplitude at many points along the basilar membrane in human cadaver ears. For practical reasons his measurements were limited to the apical end of the basilar membrane, so that he measured mainly low-frequency responses. The 'tuning curves' found by von Békésy were rather broad. The relative bandwidth was about 0.6 in the frequency range observed. This has presented a considerable problem for auditory theorists, since the observed frequency selectivity appears to be insufficient to explain either our psychoacoustically observed frequency resolving power (e.g. the ability to 'hear out' partials in a complex tone or to detect a small change in frequency), or the selectivity observed in individual neurones in the auditory nerve (see later on in this chapter). This problem will be discussed more fully in Chapters 3 and 4.

There are a number of difficulties associated with the technique used by von Békésy. Firstly, the vibration amplitudes had to be at least of the order of one wavelength of visible light, which required very high sound levels—about 140 dB SPL. It may be that the vibration of the basilar membrane is non-linear, so that it is not valid to extrapolate from these high levels to more normal sound levels. Secondly, the frequency-analysing mechanism may be physiologically vulnerable, so that the use of cadaver ears is questionable. Recent measurements of basilar membrane vibration, using different techniques, have shown that these difficulties are of considerable importance. One technique which has been extensively exploited uses an effect discovered by Mössbauer. A radioactive source of gamma rays, of very small mass and physical dimensions, is placed upon the basilar membrane. Changes in the velocity of this source, produced by motion of the basilar membrane, can be detected as a change in the wavelength of the emitted radiation. For the technically minded, this is an example of a Doppler shift. The sensitivity of this method increases with increasing frequency; at 1000 Hz a peak deflection of about 200 angstroms (Å) (1 Å is a hundred-millionth of a centimetre) can be measured, while at 10 kHz the limit is about 20 Å. This corresponds to a SPL of 70–80 dB. Thus this method has been used mainly at high frequencies, where sound levels much lower than those used by von Békésy can be utilised.

Results using this technique in live animals were reported by Johnstone and Boyle (1967), and these results have been confirmed and extended by more recent work (e.g. Johnstone, Taylor and Boyle, 1970; Rhode, 1971). Figure 1.8 compares data from Rhode

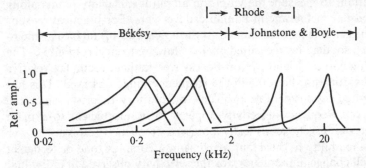

Figure 1.8 A comparison of the shapes of 'tuning curves' on the basilar membrane obtained by three different sets of workers. Each curve was obtained by measuring the amplitude of vibration at a particular point on the basilar membrane as a function of the frequency of stimulation. From Johnstone and Sellick (1972), by permission of the authors.

and Johnstone, Taylor and Boyle, with those of von Békésy. It is apparent that the 'tuning curves' obtained using the Mössbauer technique are much sharper than those of von Békésy. The slopes of his curves were 6 dB/octave on the low-frequency side and 20 dB/octave on the high-frequency side. The corresponding slopes reported by Johnstone *et al.* were 13 dB/octave and 105 dB/octave, while Rhode reported slopes of up to 200 dB/octave on the high-frequency side. It should be emphasised that these steep slopes were obtained in animals (guinea-pig and squirrel monkey) and were made in regions of the basilar membrane different from those used by von Békésy, so that direct comparison is difficult. However, the discrepancy does seem great enough to cast some doubt on von Békésy's quantitative measurements.

We mentioned above two possible difficulties associated with von Békésy's method. The first, that basilar membrane vibration may be non-linear, has been confirmed by Rhode (1971) and Rhode and Robles (1974). The non-linearity causes the peak in the pattern of vibration to flatten out at high intensities, so that a broader tuning would have been observed at the high sound levels used by von Békésy. The second, that basilar membrane responses may change after death, has been confirmed by Kohllöffel (1972, using a technique based on laser illumination of the basilar membrane) and by Rhode and Robles (1974). Not only do basilar membrane responses broaden after death, but also the non-linearity reported by Rhode disappears. Thus it appears that some aspect of the filtering action of the basilar membrane is physiologically vulnerable.

The non-linearity reported by Rhode (1971) using the Mössbauer technique is still the subject of some controversy. Rhode found that at high sound levels the peak of the 'tuning curve' increased by only 10 dB when the sound level was increased by 20 dB. Wilson and Johnstone (1972), using a method involving a capacitive probe, found that basilar membrane responses were essentially linear for sound levels up to 110 dB SPL. Unfortunately, the capacitive probe method requires the basilar membrane to be dry at the point of measurement, so that some of the fluids in the cochlea had to be drained. At the present time it is not clear whether this draining of the fluids would have been sufficient to produce the difference in results. Kohllöffel maintained a constant fluid level above the basilar membrane, in his measurements using laser light, and reported that the fluid level itself had no influence on the frequency response curves. Kohllöffel also reported that basilar membrane vibration was linear. One possible explanation for the discrepancies between the different methods is a species-specific difference; Rhode worked with the squirrel monkey, whereas Wilson and Johnstone, and Kohllöffel, used guinea-pigs. It is to be hoped that this question will soon be resolved, since the report of non-linearities has aroused considerable theoretical interest and may provide a key to the understanding of certain combination tones which occur in the auditory system (see Chapter 4).

So far we have described the responses of the basilar membrane to steady sinusoidal stimulation. While there are some disagreements about the details of the patterns of vibration, it is now beyond doubt that pure tones produce patterns with single maxima, whose positions depend upon frequency. In other words, there is a frequency-to-place conversion. The situation with other types of sounds is somewhat more complex. Consider first the case of two sinusoids, of different frequencies, presented simultaneously. The kind of pattern that will occur depends on the frequency separation of the two tones. If this is very large, then the two tones will produce two, effectively separate, patterns of vibration. Each will produce a maximum at the place on the basilar membrane which would have been excited most had that tone been presented alone. Thus the response of the basilar membrane to a low-frequency tone will be essentially unaffected by a high-frequency tone, and vice versa. In this kind of situation the basilar membrane behaves like a Fourier analyser, breaking down the complex sound into its sinusoidal components. When the two tones are relatively closer together in frequency, however, the patterns of vibration on the basilar membrane will interact, so that some points on the basilar membrane will be responding to both of the component tones. At those points the displacement on the basilar membrane as a function of time will not be sinusoidal, but will be a complex waveform resulting from the interference of the two tones. When the two tones are sufficiently close in frequency, there will no longer be a separate maximum in the pattern of vibration for each of the component tones; instead there will be a single, broader, maximum. Thus, in a sense, the basilar membrane has failed to resolve the individual frequency components. We shall see, in Chapter 3, that the frequency-resolving power of the auditory system, as observed psychoacoustically, is greater than would be expected from the patterns of vibration on the basilar membrane. Two tones an octave apart overlap considerably on the basilar membrane but are easily 'heard out' as two separate tones.

The position on the basilar membrane which is excited most by a given frequency varies approximately with the logarithm of frequency, for frequencies above 500 Hz. Further, the relative bandwidths of the patterns of vibration on the basilar membrane in response to sinusoidal stimulation are approximately constant in this frequency range. This means that the frequency separation necessary for the resolution of two tones is proportional to centre frequency. Consider how this applies to the kind of complex sound which might be produced by a musical instrument, namely a harmonic complex tone. The frequency separation between adjacent harmonics is constant (and equal to the fundamental frequency). Thus the patterns of vibration for the higher harmonics will overlap much more than those for the lower harmonics. This is illustrated schematically in Figure 1.9, which shows responses to a periodic pulse train; this stimulus is composed of harmonics which all have the same amplitude (Figure 1.3). The figure shows idealised envelopes of the patterns of excitation as a function of time (linear scale) and frequency (logarithmic scale). The lower harmonics are separated out to some extent, while at the same time the patterns of vibration corresponding to those harmonics fluctuate relatively little as a function of time. The response as a function of time to a single low harmonic is similar to the response which would have been observed

34

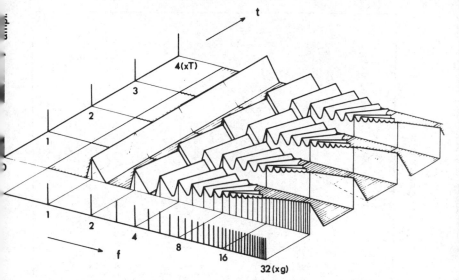

Figure 1.9   Schematic representation of the response of the basilar membrane to a series of periodic impulses. Time is plotted along the *t* axis on a linear scale; frequency (*f*) and amplitude (ampl.) scales are logarithmic. The waveform of the stimulus is indicated on the left and its spectrum is at the bottom. For the central part of the figure the frequency axis may be considered as equivalent to a position axis, indicating distance along the basilar membrane. This part of the figure shows the envelopes of the travelling wave patterns as a function of time and position. From Duifhuis (1972), by permission of the author.

if the harmonic had been presented alone. For the higher harmonics the patterns of vibration overlap to a considerable extent. The individual harmonics are no longer resolved, but the amplitude of their joint excitation pattern fluctuates strongly as a function of time. For the higher harmonics the time pattern of the response on the basilar membrane closely resembles that of the stimulus as a whole. We shall see in Chapters 3 and 4 that these factors play a crucial role in our perception of complex tones.

The response of the basilar membrane to a sudden change in sound pressure (a step function) on to a short impulse (a single click) is somewhat different. The spectra of these stimuli contain a wide range of frequencies, so that we can expect to see responses all along the basilar membrane. What happens is that a 'travelling bulge', looking like a short decaying wave train, is set up on the

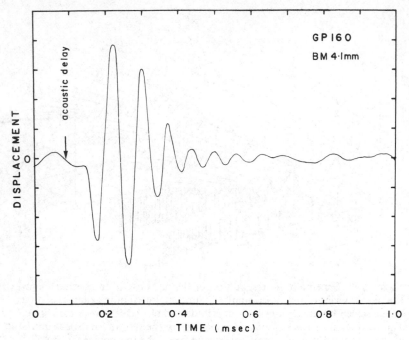

Figure 1.10 The response at a particular point on the basilar membrane to a short impulse. From Wilson and Johnstone (1972), by permission of the authors.

basilar membrane, and travels all the way along it. A number of workers have investigated the response of a single point on the basilar membrane in response to a brief click; this is called the impulse response function of that point. Figure 1.10 shows an impulse response function computed from the data of Wilson and Johnstone (1972). It looks like a damped, or decaying, sinuosidal oscillation. The frequency of this oscillation depends on which part of the basilar membrane is being studied. The basal end of the basilar membrane, which responds best to high frequencies, will show a high-frequency oscillation, while the apical end, which responds best to low frequencies, will show a low-frequency oscillation. Thus the waveform as a function of time will vary continuously with position along the basilar membrane, according to the frequency which excites that position most. We shall see in Chapter 5 that this pattern of responses affects our ability to localise sounds of a transient character.

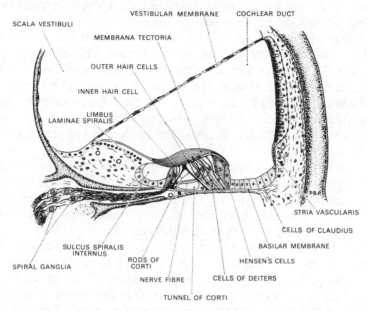

Figure 1.11   Cross-section of the cochlea, showing the organ of Corti. The actual receptors are the hair cells lying on either side of the tunnel of Corti. From Hamilton, *Textbook of Human Anatomy*, The Macmillan Press (1976).

So far we have been concerned with the mechanical responses of the basilar membrane to sound stimulation. We have seen that the basilar membrane acts as a kind of spectrum analyser, or Fourier analyser, but with a limited resolving power. Let us consider how the information about frequency, amplitude and time which is carried in the vibration patterns of the basilar membrane is converted or coded into neural signals in the auditory nervous system. Attached to the basilar membrane are hair cells, which form part of a structure called the organ of Corti (see Figure 1.11). The hair cells are divided into two groups by an arch known as the tunnel of Corti. Those on the side of the arch closest to the outside of the cochlea are known as outer hair cells, and are arranged in three rows. The hair cells on the other side of the arch form a single row, and are known as inner hair cells. There are about 25000 outer hair cells, each with about 140 hairs protruding from it, while there are about 3500 inner hair cells, each with about 40 hairs. The tectorial membrane, which is relatively stiff, lies above the hairs, and it is not at the present time clear whether the hairs are actually embedded in the tectorial membrane or whether they just rest against it. When the basilar membrane moves, this causes the hair cells to be deformed. This deformation is greater for the outer hair cells than for the inner hair cells, because the relative motion between the basilar membrane and the tectorial membrane is greater for the former. It is the deformation of the hair cells that initiates neural activity in the nerve cells connected to them. Thus the hair cells act to transduce mechanical movements into neural activity.

There are many details of the transduction process which remain poorly understood. It has been suggested that the two types of hair cells respond differently to different types of shearing motions between the basilar membrane and the tectorial membrane (see Tonndorf, 1970). More recently it has been suggested (Dallos *et al.*, 1972; Billone and Raynor, 1973) that the electrical potentials produced by the outer hair cells are proportional to the displacement of the basilar membrane, while the potentials produced by the inner hair cells are proportional to the velocity of the basilar membrane. There is general agreement that the outer hair cells have greater sensitivities than inner hair cells (i.e. that they respond at lower sound levels), and that they are more easily damaged by intense sounds. It is also possible that, because of their different modes of responding, the frequency selectivities of the inner and outer hair cells may differ (Billone and Raynor, 1973). The way in which the inner and outer hair cells are innervated is also a subject of debate. According to Spoendlin (1970), 10 per cent of auditory nerve fibres originate from outer hair cells and 90 per cent from inner hair cells. If this were the case, we might expect that there would be two distinct sets of auditory neurones with differing properties. This was once thought to be the case with respect to thresholds (Tasaki, 1954), but more recent evidence has not confirmed this (see Kiang, 1968, and the following section). Research in this area is actively continuing, but at the moment we must leave these questions in doubt.

1.4 NEURAL RESPONSES IN THE AUDITORY NERVE

Most of the recent studies of activity in the auditory nerve have used electrodes with very fine tips, known as microelectrodes. These record the nerve impulses, or spikes in single auditory nerve fibres (often called single units). Three general results have emerged, which seem to hold for most mammals. Firstly, the fibres show background or spontaneous firing in the absence of sound stimulation. Spontaneous firing rates range from close to 0 per second up to about 150 per second. Secondly, the fibres respond better to some frequencies than to others; they show frequency selectivity. Finally, the fibres show phase-locking; neural firings tend to occur at a particular phase of the stimulating waveform, so that there is a temporal regularity in the firing pattern of a neurone in response to a periodic stimulus. We will consider the last two factors in more detail.

The frequency selectivity of a single nerve fibre is often illustrated by a tuning curve, which shows the cell's threshold as a function of frequency. The curve is obtained by determining the lowest level of a sinusoid for which the experimenter, by auditory and visual monitoring of the activity in the fibre, can detect a change in activity of the fibre. The stimuli are usually tone bursts, rather than continuous tones, so that changes in activity are more easily detected. The frequency at which the threshold of the fibre is lowest is called the characteristic frequency (CF). Some typical tuning curves are presented in Figure 1.12. It may be seen that, on the logarithmic frequency scale used, the tuning curves are generally steeper on the high-frequency side than on the low-frequency one, especially for fibres with low CFs. At higher CFs the tuning curves become steeper and also more symmetrical. It is generally assumed that the frequency selectivity in single auditory nerve fibres occurs because those fibres are responding to activity in restricted regions of the basilar membrane. In other words, a single nerve fibre is assumed to derive its output from a particular part of the basilar membrane. This supposition is supported by the finding that CFs are distributed in an orderly manner in the auditory nerve. Fibres with high CFs are found in the periphery of the nerve bundle, and there is an orderly decrease in CF towards the centre of the nerve bundle (Kiang *et al.*, 1965). This kind of organisation is known as tonotopic organisation, and indicates that the place representation of frequency along the basilar membrane is preserved as a place representation in the auditory nerve. One problem in interpreting tuning curves is that their slopes are generally steeper than the corresponding slopes for patterns of vibration on the basilar membrane. This problem is discussed more fully in Chapter 3.

In order to provide a description of the characteristics of single

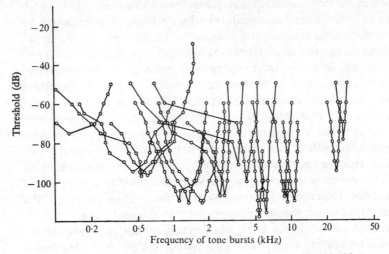

Figure 1.12 A sample of tuning curves (frequency-threshold curves) of single fibres in the auditory nerve of anaesthetised cats. The thresholds of the units as a function of frequency (logarithmic scale) are plotted on a decibel scale with arbitrary reference level. From Kiang *et al.* (1965), by permission of the author and M.I.T. Press.

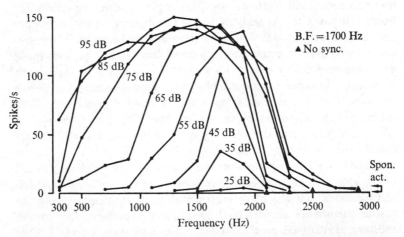

Figure 1.13 Iso-intensity contours for a single fibre in the auditory nerve of an anaesthetised squirrel monkey. Note that the frequency producing maximal firing varies as a function of level. From Rose *et al.* (1971), by permission of the authors.

fibres at levels above threshold, iso-rate contours can be plotted. To determine an iso-rate contour, the intensity of sinusoidal stimulation required to produce a predetermined firing rate in the neurone is plotted as a function of frequency. The resulting curves are generally similar in shape to tuning curves. An alternative method is to record firing rates at equal sound levels as a function of tone frequency. The resulting curves (iso-intensity contours) generally vary in shape according to the sound level chosen, and differ considerably from tuning curves (see Figure 1.13). The interpretation of iso-intensity contours is difficult, because their shape will depend upon how the rate of firing of the nerve fibre varies with intensity; this is not usually a linear function (see below). However, it is of interest that for some fibres the frequency producing maximal firing varies as a function of level. This poses some problems for one of the theories of pitch perception which will be discussed in Chapter 4.

Figure 1.14 shows how the rate of discharge of an auditory nerve fibre changes as a function of stimulus level. The stimulus was a con-tinuous tone at the CF of the unit. The general shape of the curve is typical of most auditory nerve fibres, although there is considerable variability in both the spontaneous firing rate and the maximum firing rate. Notice that above a certain sound level the neurone no longer responds to increases in sound level with an increase in firing rate; the neurone is said to be saturated. For the cat the saturation level is within about 40 dB of threshold. It is not entirely clear whether this relatively narrow 'dynamic range' is typical of other species, but if it is, then this poses severe difficulties for theories of how loudness is coded in the auditory nerve. These difficulties are compounded by the fact that the range of thresholds at a given CF is quite narrow (Kiang, 1968). These problems are discussed more fully in Chapter 2.

Although the technique of recording from single auditory neurones has provided very valuable evidence about the coding of sounds in the auditory system, it is lacking in one very fundamental respect: it does not tell us anything about the pattern of neural responses over different auditory neurones, or about possible interactions or mutual dependencies in the firing patterns of different auditory neurones. Although some attempts have been made to measure from more than one neurone simultaneously, for the most part we can only use indirect methods to find out about the total pattern of neural activity in response to a given sound. Imagine that we present (to an animal) a moderately intense pure tone of a particular

41

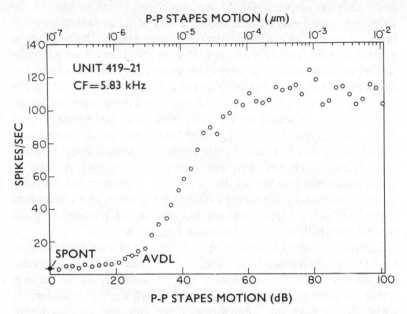

Figure 1.14 An example of how the discharge rate of a single auditory nerve fibre varies as a function of stimulus level, for a continuous stimulating tone at the CF of the neurone. The threshold of the neurone is the lowest sound level at which there is a detectable change in firing rate and is indicated by the letters AVDL (audio-visual detection level). Above a certain sound level increases in level do not produce increases in firing rate; the neurone is saturated. The range of levels between threshold and saturation is known as the 'dynamic range' and is typically 30–40 dB. The sound level is specified in dB with an arbitrary reference level. The level at the point marked AVDL corresponds to about 2 dB SPL. From Kiang (1968), by permission of the author.

frequency, say 1 kHz. We know from measurements of the responses of single neurones that this will produce a high level of activity in neurones whose characteristic frequencies (CFs) are close to 1 kHz. We also know that in units of higher and lower CFs the amount of activity (or rate of firing) will be less. If we know the tuning curve for a unit of a given CF, we can work out the amount by which the level of the tone we have presented exceeds the threshold of that unit. If we also know the function relating intensity to firing rate, we can then deduce the firing rate of the unit in response to the tone. By doing this for each CF we can work out the function relating

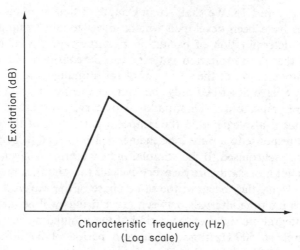

Figure 1.15 A schematic and idealised representation of the 'excitation pattern' evoked by a pure tone. The pattern represents the effective level of the stimulus in dB at each characteristic frequency.

average firing rate to CF. Such a function is called an 'excitation pattern'.

Unfortunately, there are several problems associated with this approach. Firstly, it is very laborious. Secondly, it assumes that the firing rate of a neurone depends only on the amount by which the level of the tone exceeds the threshold for the unit, and not on the frequency of the tone in relation to the CF of the unit. This does not accord very well with the experimental data. Thirdly, both spontaneous and maximum firing rates vary considerably even in neurones with similar CFs. Thus at best we could only represent what was happening in an 'average' neurone at a given CF. This last problem can be partially overcome by representing excitation patterns in a different way; instead of determining the amount of neural activity at each CF, we determine what the level of a pure tone with frequency equal to that CF would have to be in order to produce an equal amount of neural activity. Thus the excitation pattern becomes a representation of the effective amount of excitation produced by a stimulus as a function of CF, and is plotted as effective level (in dB) against CF. Normally the CF is plotted on a logarithmic scale, roughly in accord with the way that frequency appears to be represented on the basilar membrane. An idealised excitation pattern is shown in Figure 1.15. We shall see in Chapter 3 that psychoacoustic techniques have been developed which, given certain assumptions, allow the determination of excitation patterns represented in this way, and that such excitation patterns can be considered as an internal representation of the spectrum of the stimulus.

So far we have described only the changes in *rate* of firing which occur in response to a given stimulus. However, information about the stimulus is also carried in the temporal patterning of the neural firings. In response to a pure tone the nerve firings tend to be phase-locked or synchronised to the stimulating waveform. A given nerve fibre does not necessarily fire on every cycle of the stimulus, but when firings do occur, they occur at the same phase of the waveform each time. Thus the time intervals between nerve firings will be (approximately) integral multiples of the period of the stimulating waveform. For example, a 500 Hz tone will have a period of 2 milliseconds (2 ms), so that the intervals between nerve firings might be 2 ms, or 4 ms, or 6 ms, or 8 ms, etc. In general, the nerve does not fire in a completely regular manner, so that there will not be exactly 500, or 250 or 125 spikes per second. However, information about the period of the stimulating waveform is carried unambiguously in the temporal pattern of firing of a single neurone, and if we consider the responses over an ensemble of fibres, then there will be some nerve spikes on every cycle of the stimulus. Phase-locking is just what we would expect to occur as a result of the transduction process; when the basilar membrane moves upwards, towards the tectorial membrane, the hair cells are bent and a neural response is initiated. No response will occur when the basilar membrane moves downwards. Thus nerve firings tend to occur on a positive deflection of the basilar membrane produced by the rarefaction phase of the signal.

One way to demonstrate phase-locking in a single auditory nerve fibre is to plot a histogram of the time intervals between successive nerve firings. Several such interspike interval histograms are shown in Figure 1.16, for a neurone with a characteristic frequency (CF) of 1.6 kHz. For each of the different stimulating frequencies (from 0.408 to 2.3 kHz in this case) the intervals between nerve spikes lie predominantly at integral multiples of the period of the stimulating tone. These intervals are indicated by dots below each abscissa. Thus, although the neurone does not fire on every cycle of the stimulus, the distribution of time intervals between nerve firings depends closely on the frequency of the stimulating waveform.

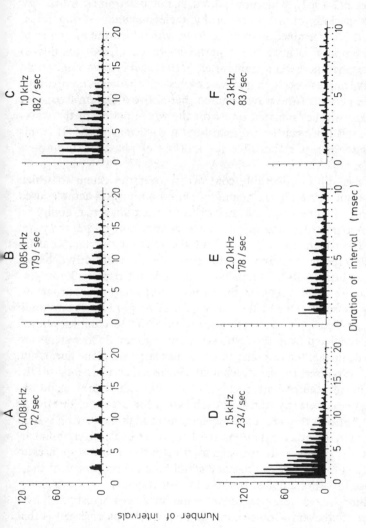

Figure 1.16 Interspike interval histograms for a single auditory neurone (in the squirrel monkey) with a CF of 1.6 kHz. Tone frequency and mean response rate in spikes per second are indicated above each histogram. All tones were at 80 dB SPL and of duration 1 s. Notice that the time scales in E and F differ from those in A to D. From Rose *et al.* (1968), by permission of the authors.

Phase-locking does not occur over the whole range of audible frequencies. The upper frequency limit seems to lie at about 4–5 kHz (Rose *et al.*, 1967). This upper limit is not determined by the refractory periods of neurones or by their maximum firing rates. Rather it is determined by the precision with which the initiation of a nerve impulse is linked to a particular phase of the stimulus. It turns out that there is a certain 'jitter' in the exact instant of initiation of a nerve impulse. At high frequencies this jitter becomes comparable with the period of the waveform, so that above a certain frequency the spikes will be 'smeared out' over the whole period of the waveform, instead of occurring primarily at a particular phase. It is this smearing which is responsible for the loss of phase-locking above 4–5 kHz.

There is still considerable controversy over the extent to which information carried in the timing of neural impulses is actually used in perceptual processes. Most workers accept that our ability to localise sounds depends in part on a comparison of the temporal information from the two ears, but the relevance of temporal information in masking and in pitch perception is still hotly debated. These problems will be discussed more fully in Chapters 3 and 4.

So far we have discussed the responses of auditory neurones to single pure tones. One of the reasons for using pure tones as stimuli is that, in many physical systems, the response to complex stimuli may be predicted from the responses to pure tones. Such systems are said to be linear; the response to a complex stimulus is the linear sum of the responses to the sinusoidal (Fourier) components of the stimulus (see the end of Section 1.2). Although neural responses themselves are clearly non-linear (showing, for example, thresholds and saturation), they sometimes behave as though the driving system were linear. In other situations the behaviour is clearly non-linear, so that it is necessary to investigate directly the neural responses to complex stimuli, if we are to understand how the properties of these complex stimuli are coded in the auditory system.

Auditory nerve responses to two tones have been investigated by a number of workers. One striking finding which has emerged is that the tone-driven activity of a single fibre in response to one tone can be suppressed by the presence of a second tone. This has been called two-tone inhibition (Sachs and Kiang, 1968), although the term 'two-tone suppression' is now generally preferred. Typically the phenomenon is investigated by presenting a tone at, or close to, the CF of a neurone. A second tone is then presented, its frequency and intensity are varied, and the effects of this on the response of the neurone are noted. The suppressing tone usually has its greatest effect at frequencies slightly above or below the area of the unit's excitatory response to a single tone. The suppression effects begin and cease very rapidly, within a few milliseconds of the onset and termination of the second tone (Arthur, Pfeiffer and Suga, 1971). Thus it is unlikely that the suppression is established through any elaborate neural interconnections. It is possible that they are related to non-linear mechanical events on the basilar membrane (Legouix, Remond and Greenbaum, 1973; Rhode and Robles, 1974).

The effects of two-tone stimulation on temporal patterns of neural firing have also been studied. For tones which are non-harmonically related Hind *et al.* (1967) found that discharges may be phase-locked to one tone, or the other, or to both tones simultaneously. Which of these occurs is determined by the intensities of the two tones and their frequencies in relation to the 'response area' of the fibre. When phase-locking occurs to only one tone of a pair, each of which is effective when acting alone, the temporal structure of the response may be indistinguishable from that which occurs when that tone is presented alone. Further, the discharge rate may be similar to the value produced by that tone alone. Thus the dominant tone appears to 'capture' the response of the neurone. We will discuss in Chapter 3 the possibility that this 'capture effect' underlies the masking of one sound by another.

Brugge *et al.* (1969) investigated auditory nerve responses to pairs of tones with simple frequency ratios (i.e. harmonically related tones). They drew the following conclusions: (1) auditory nerve fibres are excited by deflections of the cochlear partition (basilar membrane) if only one direction; (2) the discharges occur at times which correspond to the elevations of the stimulating waveform; (3) the effective stimulating waveform can be approximated by addition of the component sinusoids, although the required amplitude and phase relations usually cannot be taken directly from the actual stimulus parameters. The results of Brugge *et al.* indicate that interactions between two tones may take place even when their frequencies are quite widely separated (frequency ratios between the two tones of up to 7:1 were used).

Javel (1974) investigated the responses in single auditory neurones to stimuli consisting of three successive high harmonics of a complex

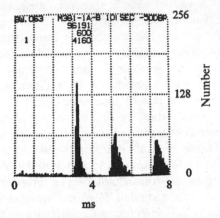

Figure 1.17. A post-stimulus time (PST) histogram showing the number of nerve spikes occurring in response to a click, presented repeatedly, as a function of the time delay from the instant of presentation of the click. The time interval between peaks in the histogram corresponds to the reciprocal of the CF of the neurone (540 Hz). From Kiang *et al.* (1965), by permission of the author and M.I.T. Press.

tone. He showed that a portion of the neural activity in the neurones responding to the component frequencies was phase-locked to the overall repetition rate of the stimulus (equal to the absent fundamental frequency). We will discuss in Chapter 4 the possibility that such temporal coding is responsible for the pitch of complex tones.

The responses of auditory neurones to clicks are closely related to the corresponding patterns of vibration which occur on the basilar membrane (see Section 1.3). Such responses are often plotted in the form of post-stimulus time (PST) histograms. To determine a PST histogram the click is presented many times, and the numbers of neural impulses occurring at various times after the instant of click presentation are counted. These are then plotted in the form of a histogram, with the instant of click presentation being taken as time zero (see Figure 1.17). It may be seen that spikes tend to occur at certain preferred intervals after the presentation of the click, as indicated by the peaks in the histogram. The multiple peaks presumably occur because the response of the basilar membrane to a click is a damped or decaying oscillation (see Figure 1.10). Nerve firings will tend to occur at a particular phase of this damped oscillation. The time intervals between the peaks correspond to the CF of the neurone.

48

If the polarity of the click is reversed (e.g. from rarefaction to condensation) the pattern is shifted in time, so that peaks now appear where dips were located. The latency of the first peak is shortest for rarefaction clicks, again indicating that the excitation of hair cells occurs when the basilar membrane is deflected towards the tectorial membrane. These factors are particularly relevant to our ability to locate sounds of a transient character (see Chapter 5).

1.5 NEURAL RESPONSES AT HIGHER LEVELS IN THE AUDITORY SYSTEM

In the visual system it is known that neurones respond preferentially to certain features of the stimulus, such as lines of particular orientation, movement, colour, etc. There seems to be a hierarchy of specialised neural detectors (sometimes called feature detectors), ranging from centre-surround units to hypercomplex cells (Hubel and Wiesel, 1968). The information in the optic nerve is recorded and processed at different points in the visual system, so that the responses of cortical units are very different from those in the optic nerve.

Much the same thing seems to happen in the auditory system, except that it is much less clear what the crucial features of the stimulus are which will produce responses from a given neurone, or set of neurones. In addition, the anatomy of the auditory system is exceedingly complex, so that many of the neural pathways within and between the various nuclei in the auditory system have yet to be investigated in detail. It is beyond the scope of this book to give more than the briefest description of recent research on the neurophysiology of higher centres in the auditory system. We will content ourselves with describing some properties of cortical neurones, and will introduce other data later in the book, when they have some relevance to the mechanism or process under discussion. Some of the more important neural centres, or nuclei in the auditory pathway are illustrated in Figure 1.18.

It is likely that the cortex is concerned with analysing more complex aspects of stimuli than simple pitch or loudness. Many cortical neurones will not respond to steady pure tones at all, and the tuning properties of those which do respond to pure tones tend to differ from those found in primary auditory neurones. Abeles and Goldstein (1972) found three different types of tuning properties: narrow,

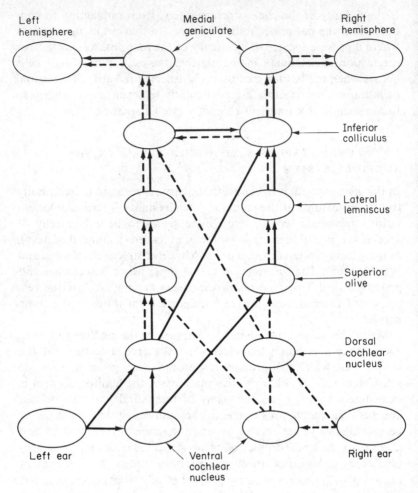

Figure 1.18 An illustration of the most important pathways and nuclei from the ear to the auditory cortex. The nuclei illustrated are located in the brain stem.

broad and multi-range (responding to a number of preferred frequencies). They considered that this suggested a hierarchical organisation, with several narrow-range units converging on one multi-range unit. There is some dispute whether the tonotopic organisation which is found at lower levels in the auditory system persists at the cortex. Merzenich, Knight and Roth (1973a), using characteristic frequency determinations in the anaesthetised cat, reported a highly ordered tonotopic organisation; the CF changes in an orderly way according to the place of penetration of the electrode. On the other hand, Evans (1968), using unanaesthetised, unrestrained cats, found only a very general trend in the location of unit CFs. He considered that what little trend there was represented a residuum of anatomical arrangement from sub-cortical levels, rather than a property which had a function significance for frequency analysis. A number of studies have indicated that anaesthetics do considerably alter the responses of cortical neurones, so that data obtained using anaesthetics must be interpreted with considerable caution.

Evans (1968), using mostly unanaesthetised cats, has reported that 20 per cent of cortical neurones respond only to complex stimuli such as clicks, bursts of noise or 'kissing' sounds. Ten per cent of those neurones which would respond to tonal stimuli would only do so if the tone frequency was changing. Whitfield and Evans (1965) reported that frequency-modulated tones were very effective stimuli for the majority of neurones responding to tones. Many neurones exhibited responses which were preferential to certain directions of frequency change. These neurones have been called 'frequency sweep detectors'. Some neurones respond preferentially to particular rates of modulation or to particular rates of frequency sweep.

For other neurones repetition rate and duration of steady tonal stimuli were critical parameters. Seventeen per cent of all units studied responded only to the onset of a tonal stimulus, while 10 per cent responded only to the termination and 2 per cent responded to both onset and termination. Over 50 per cent of neurones were preferentially or specifically sensitive to particular locations of the sound source. This general finding has been confirmed and extended by Brugge and Merzenich (1973) for restraining, unanaesthetised monkeys. They found that many units were sensitive to interaural (between the ears) time or intensity differences. At low frequencies spike count was a periodic function of interaural time delay. In several penetrations neighbouring cells were most sensitive to the same interaural delay. Some cells were sensitive to small interaural shifts in sound pressure levels over a range of about 20 dB. We shall see in Chapter 5 that the features of the stimuli to which these cells are responsive are crucial in our ability to localise sounds.

Wollberg and Newman (1972) investigated the responses of cortical neurones in awake squirrel monkeys to recorded species-

4-2

specific vocalisations. They found some cells which responded with temporally complex patterns of neural firing to many different vocalisations. Other cells responded to only one call, with simpler patterns of firing. Deletion of short segments of the calls revealed that specific segments of the calls are responded to by different cells, but that the relationship between the response and the temporal characteristics of the call is a complex one, involving preceding portions of the call. The results suggest that cortical cells are specialised for the detection of certain acoustic features which occur in monkey cells. At the present time we have no way of knowing whether there are similar neurones in humans which are specialised for the detection and analysis of specific speech sounds, although there do appear to be areas in the human brain which are specialised for the perception of speech (see Chapter 6).

2

Loudness, Adaptation and Fatigue

2.1 INTRODUCTION

The human ear is remarkable both in terms of its absolute sensitivity and in terms of the range of intensities to which it can respond. The loudest sound we can hear without damaging our ears has a level about 140 dB above the faintest sound we can detect. This corresponds to a ratio of powers of 100 000 000 000 000:1. One aim of this chapter is to discuss the possible ways in which such a range could be coded. A second aim is to discuss how loudness of sounds depends upon frequency and intensity, and to relate this to the way in which these sounds are processed.

A problem which arises in studying the loudness of sounds, particularly when these are complex or of a transient nature, is that loudness is a subjective quantity, and as such cannot be measured directly. This problem has been tackled in a number of different ways: sometimes subjects are asked to match the loudness of a sound to some standard comparison stimulus (often a 1000 Hz tone); in other experiments subjects are asked to rate loudness on a numerical scale, a technique known as magnitude estimation. As we shall see, there are problems associated with each of these methods.

A third area of discussion will be that of loudness adaptation, fatigue and damage risk. In general, adaptation and fatigue in the auditory system are much less marked than in the visual system, and the effects also have different time courses. In certain types of deafness adaptation effects become more marked. We will discuss how this, and the phenomenon of recruitment (see below), can be used in the differential diagnosis of hearing disorders.

53

2.2 ABSOLUTE THRESHOLDS

A large number of workers have determined absolute thresholds for pure tones as a function of frequency. Quite large discrepancies are apparent in the results. At least part of the variability is attributable to differences in what is being measured. Some experimenters have delivered tones via headphones, measuring what is called minimum audible pressure (MAP). The physical values of the sound pressures have been determined by calibrating the headphones using 'artificial ears', or by using a microphone with a probe tube attached, so that sound pressures either at the entrance to the meatus or at the eardrum could be measured. Other workers have delivered tones via loudspeakers, measuring the minimum audible field (MAF). Sound pressures were determined either at the entrance to the meatus, or at the eardrum, or at the centre of the position which had been occupied by the head, the listener having been removed from the sound field.

A typical set of results for MAP are shown in Figure 2.1. These were obtained by Dadson and King (1952), using a sample of 198 ears, with sound pressures measured at two positions close to the entrance to the meatus. The distribution of thresholds for the same group of listeners at four different frequencies is shown in Figure 2.2. Although the subjects were 'otologically normal', with ages between 18 and 25 years, it is clear that there is a large variability among different observers. Part of this may be attributable to criterion differences; the proportion of 'yes' responses by the subject will be affected by his willingness to respond to minimal sensory evidence (see Section 3.7). However, the range of thresholds is probably much too large to be explained in this way. Tumarkin (1972) has suggested that the majority of the ears tested in this sample may have been biologically subnormal, and he cites evidence from Bredberg (1968) showing that the number of hair cells in the inner ear is diminishing almost from the day we are born. It is certainly puzzling that a considerable number of subjects had thresholds 20 dB or more below the mean.

The general shape of the frequency–threshold curve (often called the audiogram) is now well established. We are most sensitive to frequencies in the range 1000–5000 Hz, while thresholds increase rapidly at very high and very low frequencies. At least part of our sensitivity to middle frequencies derives from the action of the pinna

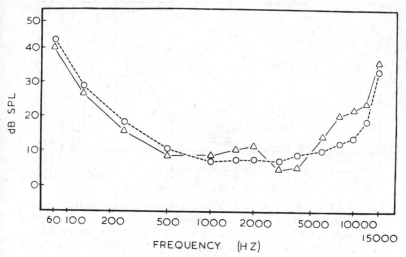

Figure 2.1   The minimum audible sound level as a function of frequency for two positions close to the entrance of the ear canal (meatus). The solid curve gives sound levels measured 0.3 cm inside the entrance to the meatus, and the dashed curve levels measured 0.7 cm outside the entrance to the meatus. Redrawn from Dadson and King (1952), by permission of the authors and the director of the National Physical Laboratory, UK.

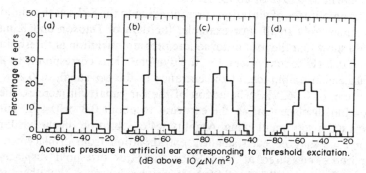

Figure 2.2   The distribution of sound levels at threshold for 198 ears at four frequencies. Redrawn from Dadson and King (1952), by permission of the authors and the director of the National Physical Laboratory, UK.

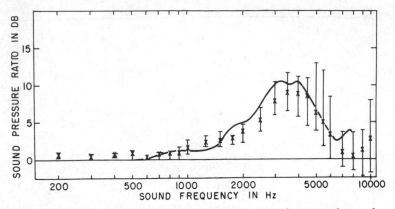

Figure 2.3 The transformation in sound pressure between the eardrum and the entrance to the ear canal. Crosses indicate the means, vertical bars the interquartile ranges. The solid line reproduces earlier data of Wiener and Ross (1946). From Djupesland and Zwislocki (1972), by permission of the authors.

and ear canal. Figure 2.3, from Djupesland and Zwislocki (1972), shows the sound pressure transformation between the eardrum and a point 1 cm outside the tragus (the small projection at the entrance to the ear canal). The outer ear enhances the sound pressure at the eardrum for frequencies in the range 1–9 kHz, with a maximum enhancement at 3 kHz of about 15 dB.

The amplitudes of vibration corresponding to the SPLs at threshold are remarkably small. For example, the data of Dadson and King (1952) show that the root mean square pressure variation at threshold for a 3000 Hz tone is about 4×10^{-4} dyn/cm^2. This corresponds to a displacement amplitude, at the entrance to the ear canal, of 6.25 × 10^{-10} cm, or 0.0625 Å. The action of the ear canal will increase the threshold displacement at the eardrum to about 0.3 or 0.4 Å, but this is still a very small value. Amplitudes of vibration on the basilar membrane may be even smaller; extrapolation from displacement amplitudes measured at high SPLs indicates threshold displacements of between 0.01 and 0.05 Å. It may be, however, that there is some non-linearity in the behaviour of the basilar membrane, in which case such extrapolations are not justified (Rhode, 1971).

At low frequencies MAPs, measured under headphones, are greater than MAFs, by between 5 and 10 dB. A number of workers have shown that this is due to physiological noise of vascular origin, which is produced within the meatus when earphones are worn (Anderson and Whittle, 1971; Soderquist and Lindsey, 1972). The detectability of low-frequency tones can be shown to vary according to their temporal position within the cardiac cycle (heart-beat). The level of this low-frequency 'physiological noise' varies with the leakage of air around the headphone (this will depend in part on headband pressure), with the volume of the subject's meatus, and with the strength of his heart-beat. These sources of variance are lessened when circumaural headphones (which fit around the pinnae) rather than supra-aural headphones (which lie over and flatten the pinnae) are used. Thus circumaural earphones are preferable for use at low frequencies. However, at high frequencies these headphones are less reliable, and more difficult to calibrate than supra-aural headphones.

The highest audible frequency varies considerably with the age of the subject. Young children can often hear tones as high as 20 kHz, but for most adults threshold rises rapidly above about 15 kHz. The loss of sensitivity with increasing age (presbyacusis) is much greater at high frequencies than at low, and the variability between different observers is also greater at high frequencies. At the other end of the scale there seems to be no particular low-frequency limit to our hearing. Whittle, Collins and Robinson (1972) measured thresholds for frequencies from 50 Hz down to 3.15 Hz, and showed that their results formed a continuum with the results at higher frequencies. However, for the 3.15 Hz tone the threshold level was about 120 dB SPL! It has been suggested (Johnson and von Gierke, 1974) that sounds below about 16 Hz are not heard in the normal sense, but are detected by virtue of the distortion products (harmonics) which they produce after being transduced through the middle ear. Thus the lower frequency limit for the 'true' hearing of pure tones probably lies about 16 Hz. This is also close to the lowest frequency for which the attribute of pitch remains meaningful.

In many practical situations our ability to detect faint sounds is limited not by our absolute sensitivity to those sounds but by the level of ambient noise. In other words, detection will depend upon the masked threshold rather than the absolute threshold. In such cases the threshold as a function of frequency will depend upon the character of the ambient noise (e.g. frequency content, level, whether intermittent or continuous, etc). These problems are discussed more fully in Chapter 3.

2.3 EQUAL-LOUDNESS CONTOURS

There are many occasions on which engineers and acousticians require some subjective scale corresponding to the loudness of a sound. Since complex sounds are often analysed in terms of their individual frequency components, a useful first step is to derive such a scale for pure tones. The most direct way of doing this is to use the technique of magnitude estimation, to determine the relationship between physical intensity and judged loudness. However, the validity of this technique has been questioned, and before discussing it (Section 2.4) we will consider an alternative measure of loudness, which is not at first sight so straightforward, but which nevertheless has proved useful in practice, and which is not so controversial. The alternative is the Loudness Level, which tells us not how loud a tone is, but rather how intense a 1000 Hz tone must be in order to sound equally loud. The psychophysical task required of the subject is a judgement of equal loudness with respect to two tones of different frequency. Results are usually presented in terms of equal-loudness contours. For example, the standard reference tone might be presented at 40 dB SPL. The subject is then presented with a tone of different frequency, say 500 Hz, and is asked to adjust its intensity until it sounds as loud as the 1000 Hz 40 dB tone. The Loudness Level of the 500 Hz tone is then defined to be 40 phons.

Thus the Loudness Level of any tone is the Intensity Level (in dB SPL) of the 1000 Hz tone to which it sounds equal in loudness. The unit of Loudness Level is the phon. Some typical results are shown in Figure 2.4 (from Robinson and Dadson, 1956). This figure shows equal-loudness contours for Loudness Levels from 20 phons to 120 phons, and it also includes the absolute threshold (MAF) curve. The equal-loudness contours are of similar shape to the threshold curve, but tend to become flatter at high Loudness Levels. This means that the rate of growth of loudness differs for tones of different frequency. For example, the absolute threshold for a 100 Hz tone is about 20 dB above that for a 1000 Hz tone (thresholds at 23 and 3 dB SPL). But for the 100 phon contour the intensities are nearly the same (102 and 100 dB SPL). For the same range of loudness, from threshold to 100 phons, the intensity of the 1000 Hz tone must be increased by 97 dB, while that of the 100 Hz tone must be increased by only 79 dB. Thus the rate of growth of loudness with increase in intensity is greater for low frequencies

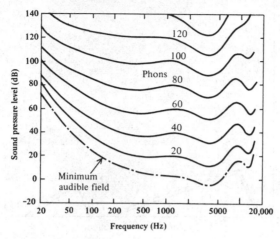

Figure 2.4 Equal-loudness contours for various loudness levels. The absolute threshold curve is also indicated. Redrawn from Robinson and Dadson (1956), by permission of the authors and the director of the National Physical Laboratory, UK.

(and to some extent for very high frequencies) than for middle frequencies.

These findings have certain implications for the reproduction of sound; the relative loudness of the different frequency components in the sound will change as a function of the overall intensity, so that unless the sounds are reproduced at the same intensity as the original, the 'tonal balance' will be altered. This is one of the reasons why human voices often sound 'boomy' when reproduced at high levels via loudspeakers; the ear becomes relatively more sensitive to low frequencies at high intensities. Conversely, at low levels we are less sensitive to the very low and very high frequencies, so that many amplifiers incorporate a 'loudness' control which boosts the bass (and to some extent the treble) at low listening levels. Such controls are not usually very effective, since they take no account of loudspeaker efficiency, size of room, etc.

The explanation for the greater rate of growth of loudness at low frequencies may lie in the way the patterns of vibration on the basilar membrane change as a function of intensity. For low frequencies the vibrations on the basilar membrane spread over a much larger area than for high frequencies (see Figure 2.5). Thus an increase in intensity will cause a change in the amount of excitation in a larger

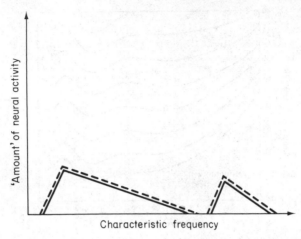

Figure 2.5 Idealised 'excitation patterns' for a low-frequency tone and a high-frequency tone, both of moderate level. An increase in level, indicated by the dashed lines, produces a change in firing rate in a greater number of neurones for the low-frequency tone than for the high-frequency tone.

number of neurones at low frequencies. If a change in loudness is signalled as a change in the total number of neural firings, then this will lead to a more rapid growth of loudness at low frequencies.

The shapes of equal-loudness contours have been used in the design of sound level meters which attempt to give an approximate measure of the loudness of complex sounds. Such meters contain weighting networks, so that the meter does not simply sum the power at all different frequencies, but rather weights the power at each frequency according to the shape of the equal-loudness contours. At low sound levels low-frequency components contribute little to the total loudness of a complex sound, so an 'A' weighting is used which reduces the contribution of low frequencies to the final meter reading. At high levels all frequencies contribute more or less equally to the loudness sensation (the equal-loudness contours being approximately flat), so that a more nearly linear weighting characteristic, the 'C' network, is used. The 'B' weighting is used for intermediate levels. Sound levels measured with these meters are usually specified in terms of the weighting used. Thus a given level might be specified as 35 dBA, meaning that the meter gave a reading of 35 dB when the 'A' weighting was used.

The sound level meters which we have described suffer from a number of problems. Firstly, they can only be reliably used with steady sounds of relatively long duration; the responses to transient sounds do not correspond to the subjective impressions of the loudness of such sounds. Secondly, they do not provide a satisfactory way of summing the loudness of components in widely separated frequency bands. As we shall see in Chapter 3, the loudness of a complex sound with a given amount of energy depends on whether that energy is contained within a narrow range of frequencies or is spread over a wide range of frequencies. Bauer, Torick and Allen (1971) have described several stages in the development of a sound level meter which attempts to overcome these problems. These stages include:

(1) The determination of equal-loudness contours for octave bands of pink noise. Such noise has constant energy in a given relative bandwidth (bandwidth divided by centre frequency), and is representative of many of the broad-band sounds encountered in everyday life.

(2) The determination of appropriate meter ballistics, so that the meter can cope with fluctuating and transient sounds.

(3) The determination of a rule for adding loudness levels in different octave bands. The rule used actually involved the arithmetic addition of loudness levels in different bands.

A loudness level meter based on these principles was evaluated by asking subjects to make judgements of the relative loudness of a variety of complex sounds and comparing their judgements with the readings given by the meter. The results indicated a considerable superiority over the conventional loudness meter.

It should not be assumed that such meters give a 'true' estimate of the loudness of a given sound. The readings obtained are closely related to the decibel scale, which is a scale of physical magnitude rather than a scale of subjective sensation (see below). Thus it would be quite wrong to say that a sound giving a reading of 80 dB was twice as loud as a sound giving a reading of 40 dB. However, the meters do enable us to roughly compare the loudness of different complex sounds. We shall discuss below some of the models which attempt to provide more satisfactory estimates of the loudness of complex sounds.

2.4 THE SCALING OF LOUDNESS

We will not attempt here to discuss in detail the methods which have been used to construct scales of loudness, and the methods which have been used to validate them. The development of scales of loudness and of other sensory dimensions has been pioneered by S. S. Stevens, and the reader is referred to his work for further details (Stevens, 1957). Stevens proposed the sone as the unit of loudness, and we will discuss briefly how a sone scale of loudness could be constructed. One sone is defined arbitrarily as the loudness of a 1000 Hz tone at 40 dB SPL. The listener is asked to adjust the level of a 1000 Hz tone until it sounds half as loud as this standard of 40 dB. This loudness is labelled 0.5 sone. Similarly, a sound that is judged to be twice as loud will have a loudness of 2 sones. By continuing this process a wide range of intensities can be explored, and intermediate points can be obtained by a method of bisection, e.g. a tone whose loudness is judged to be halfway between that of a 2 sone tone and a 4 sone tone will have a loudness of 3 sones.

On the basis of his own observations on large numbers of subjects, and using the results of other workers, Stevens suggested that loudness, as defined by the sone scale, was a power function of physical intensity: $L = kI^{0.3}$ where k is a constant depending on the subject and the units used. In other words, the loudness of a given sound will be proportional to its intensity raised to the power 0.3. A simple approximation to this is that a twofold change in loudness is equivalent to a 10 dB step.

The sone scale has been used by Zwicker and Scharf (1965), Zwicker (1958) and Stevens (1972) in models which allow the calculation of the loudness of complex sounds. We will not present these models in detail, since they are rather complicated. Although there are some differences in the models, in essence they involve the splitting of the complex stimulus into a number of frequency bands (usually $\frac{1}{3}$ octave bands), and the determination of the level in each one. The level in each band is then converted to a 'loudness' on the sone scale, using Steven's Power Law, and the loudness in each band is summed to give the total loudness.

There have been many criticisms of loudness scaling. The technique seems very susceptible to bias effects, so that results are affected by the range of stimuli presented, the first stimulus presented, the instructions to the subject, the range of permissible responses, symmetry of the response range (judgements tend to be biased towards the middle of the range available for responses), and various other factors related to experience, motivation, training, attention, etc. Very large individual differences are observed, and consistent results are only obtained by averaging many judgements of a large number of subjects. Warren (1970a) attempted to eliminate known bias effects by obtaining just a single judgement from each subject. Only those responses distributed symmetrically about the centre of the available range were considered as bias-free. He found that half-loudness corresponds to a 6 dB attenuation, rather than the 10 dB suggested by Stevens. However, considerable variability is also apparent in his data.

It is not at all clear that methods of calculating loudness using the 'psychological' sone scale give better agreement with loudness judgements than methods based on a physical analysis of the stimuli. Thus Corliss and Winzer (1964) say: 'The loudness of several complex sounds computed on the basis of Stevens' model did not agree with the results of Zwicker's model. The results were not related in any consistent way and both sets of computations were at variance with the subjects' response.' Similarly, Howes (1971) compared the loudness of broad-band noise calculated by a method similar to Zwicker's, with the loudness calculated by summing weighted intensities of sub-bands of noise and obtaining the loudness of the sum. This 'power summation' method gave better agreement with actual loudness judgements than did Zwicker's method. Carter (1972) applied five different methods in the calculation of the loudness of repeated acoustic transients. A white noise was used as a comparison stimulus. The method predicting loudness most effectively in the face of variation in rise time and repetition rate of the transients was dBA, a measure obtained using a sound level meter with 'A' weighting (see Section 2.3). This method was clearly superior to methods employing the sone scale.

At the present time there are a great many competing methods for calculating loudness, and no one method seems to be entirely successful in dealing with the great variety of sounds which are encountered in everyday life. There is certainly room for considerable scepticism when a statement such as 'Concorde is twice as loud as a Boeing 747' is made.

2.5 TEMPORAL INTEGRATION

It has been known for many years (Exner, 1876) that both absolute thresholds and the loudness of sounds depend upon duration. The studies of absolute threshold which were described earlier were all carried out with sounds, usually tone bursts, of relatively long duration, and it does appear to be the case that for durations exceeding about 500 ms threshold is independent of duration. However, for durations less than about 200 ms the sound intensity necessary for detection increases as duration decreases (remember that intensity is a measure of energy per unit time). A number of workers have investigated the relation between threshold and duration for tone pulses, over a wide range of frequencies and durations.

The early work of Hughes (1946) and Garner and Miller (1947) indicated that, over a reasonable range of durations, the ear appears to integrate the energy of the stimulus over time, in the detection of short-duration tone bursts. Ideally this would be expressed by the formula

$$I \times t = \text{constant,} \qquad (2.1)$$

where I is the threshold intensity for a tone pulse of duration t. In other words, the threshold would depend only on the total amount of energy in the stimulus and not on how that energy was distributed over time. In practice the results are fitted better by the expression

$$(I - I_L) \times t = I_L \times \tau = \text{constant,} \qquad (2.2)$$

where I_L is the threshold intensity for a long-duration tone pulse and τ is a constant representing the 'integration time' of the auditory system. Notice that in this formula it is not the product of time and intensity which is constant, but the product of time and the amount by which the intensity exceeds the value I_L. Garner and Miller interpreted I_L as the minimum intensity which is an effective stimulus for the ear. They assumed that only intensities above this minimum value are integrated linearly by the ear.

Plomp and Bouman (1959) suggested an alternative way of accounting for the experimental results. They put forward the hypothesis that switching on a tone pulse of intensity I results in a sensory effect S that approaches its end value asymptotically according to an exponential function, this end value being proportional to I. Detection occurs when S exceeds a critical value S_0.

According to this hypothesis the relation between S and I is given by

$$S = kI(1 - e^{-t/\tau}), \tag{2.3}$$

where t is the time after the start of the pulse, k is a constant and τ is a time constant which determines the rate of increase of S. Detection would occur when

$$kI(1 - e^{-t/\tau}) = S_0. \tag{2.4}$$

When t is much less than τ, Equation (2.4) becomes identical with Equation (2.2), but at longer durations there are differences. On the basis of a number of experiments, Plomp and Bouman concluded that their hypothesis gave a better description of the data than other hypotheses thus far used (including that of Miller and Garner). However, the data deviate from the predictions of their hypothesis at very short durations.

Plomp and Bouman found that the time constant of integration varies according to frequency, being around 375 ms at 250 Hz and 150 ms at 8000 Hz. Other workers have also found time constants which vary with frequency (e.g. Watson and Gengel, 1968), although the actual values of the time constants have not always been in agreement. On the other hand, Olsen and Carhart (1966) found for frequencies of 250, 1000 and 4000 Hz that changes in threshold with stimulus duration were similar for all stimuli, while Bilger and Feldman (1968) reported that results depend upon the particular method chosen to measure temporal integration.

The limits of complete energy integration have been studied using tone pulses of various durations but with equal energy (Green, Birdsall and Tanner, 1957). In theory, complete integration would lead to constant detectability. Green and co-workers used as their measure of detectability the quantity d', which is derived from the theory of signal detection (see Section 3.7). They found that detectability was generally constant over the range of durations from 15 to 150 ms, but fell off for durations smaller or greater than this (see Figure 2.6). A similar 'plateau' was found by Sheeley and Bilger (1964), although the plateau occurred at longer durations for low frequencies (250 Hz) and shorter durations at high frequencies (4000 Hz). The fall in detectability at longer durations is in line with previous studies, indicating that there is a limit to the time over which the ear can integrate energy (or a lower limit to the intensity which can be effectively integrated). The fall in detectability at very short durations may be connected with the inevitable spread of

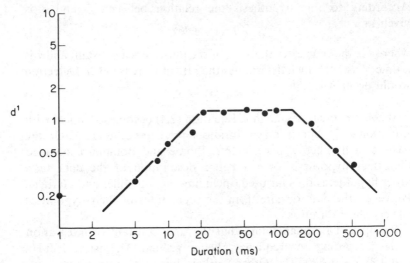

Figure 2.6 The mean detectability of (d') of equal energy tone bursts of frequency 1 kHz as a function of duration. Note the range of durations over which detectability is roughly constant. From Stephens (1973), by permission of the author.

energy over frequency which occurs for signals of short duration (see Section 1.2). It may be that energy can only be integrated when it falls within a fairly narrow range of frequencies and that this range is exceeded for signals of very short duration. This idea is closely connected with the concept of the critical band, which is discussed in Chapter 3.

The pattern of results found for equal energy signals—a plateau of detectability for durations from about 15 to 150 ms, with a fall in detectability outside this range—has been found both for absolute thresholds and for masked thresholds, when the tone pulses are presented against a noise background. Stephens (1973) investigated the effect of overall intensity (maintaining a constant signal-to-noise ratio) and found two effects of level in different parts of the range of stimulus durations. Firstly, the very-short-duration stimuli (less than 20 ms) were less detectable at intermediate levels (60 dB) than at higher or lower levels. Secondly, the time constant of integration, or the point at which detectability begins to decrease at long durations, becomes shorter with increasing overall level. The explanation for these effects is not clear, although the second effect may be related to the increased rate of adaptation which is found in the cochlear nerve and cochlear nucleus with increasing stimulus intensity (Zwislocki, 1969).

The effect of duration on loudness has also been measured extensively, but the results show considerable variability except for a general agreement that, at a given intensity, loudness increases with duration. Boone (1973) required subjects to match the loudness of tone bursts to that of a continuous reference tone. He found that for a frequency of 1 kHz the loudness was related to the total energy of the burst. He also found that the off-time between repeated bursts had an effect, and that this effect was frequency-dependent. Stephens (1974) investigated the loudness of equal-energy tone bursts of various durations using two different techniques. In the first, subjects were required to give a numerical estimate of the loudness of tone bursts in relation to a standard which was presented initially and stated to have a loudness of 100. In the second, subjects were required to adjust the intensity of a fixed-duration stimulus so that its loudness matched that of the tone burst being judged. Stephens also investigated the effect of different sets of instructions. He found that in most cases there was a plateau for a particular range of durations, indicating that equal energy means equal loudness, but that experimental paradigm and the exact wording of instructions did affect the results. One reason for this is that listeners find it difficult to separate the loudness and duration aspects of the stimuli in making their judgements. With both techniques the plateau tended to occur at shorter durations for higher frequencies. The influence of duration in loudness is discussed further in Chapter 3.

2.6 THE DETECTION OF INTENSITY CHANGES AND THE CODING OF LOUDNESS

The smallest detectable change in intensity has been measured for many different types of stimuli by a variety of methods. Harris (1963) called the two principal methods loudness modulation and loudness memory. Riesz (1928) used the former method, in which periodic smooth intensity changes are introduced into the signal (Riesz did this by mixing the outputs of two oscillators at slightly different frequencies) and the smallest detectable change in intensity is determined. The second technique involves the presentation of two stimuli, the observer being required to judge which is the more

5-2

intense, i.e. the two-alternative forced-choice procedure is used. The intensity DL is usually defined as that intensity difference which produces 75 per cent correct responses.

Harris (1963) has presented extensive data for both types of task. Since then a large number of papers have appeared giving intensity DLs for a variety of stimuli. Although there are some minor discrepancies in the experimental results, the general trend is quite clear. For wide-band noise, or for bands of noise of restricted frequency range, the smallest detectable intensity change is approximately a constant fraction of the intensity of the stimulus. If I is the intensity of a noise band, and ΔI is the smallest detectable change in intensity, then $\Delta I/I$ is roughly constant. In other words, Weber's Law holds. If we express the smallest detectable change in decibels, i.e. as $10 \log [(\Delta I + I)/I]$, then this, too, will be constant. Thus the just-detectable change in level, expressed in decibels, will be constant, regardless of the absolute intensity, and for wide-band noise has a value of about 0.5–1 dB (Rodenburg, 1972). This holds from about 20 dB above threshold to 100 dB above threshold (Miller, 1947).

For pure tones the situation is somewhat different. Riesz's data for modulated tones, and data from a number of other workers using pulsed tones (2-AFC task), shows that Weber's Law does not hold (see, for example, Viemeister, 1972). Instead it is found that if ΔI (in dB) is plotted against I (also in dB), a straight line is obtained with a slope of about 0.9. Thus discrimination, as measured by the Weber fraction, improves at high levels. This has been termed the 'near miss' to Weber's Law. The data of Riesz for loudness modulation show a DL of 1.5 dB at 20 dB SL, 0.7 dB at 40 dB SL, and 0.3 dB at 80 dB SL (all at 1000 Hz).

Let us consider the implications of these findings in terms of the physiological coding of intensity in the auditory system. The two major factors which we have to explain are: (1) the auditory system is capable of detecting changes in intensity for a range of intensities of at least 100 dB; and (2) Weber's Law holds for the discrimination of bursts of noise but not for pure tones.

For many years it was thought that there were groups of auditory nerve fibres with widely differing thresholds (see, for example, Tasaki, 1954). This loudness could be coded simply in terms of which fibres were active. However, more recent data, obtained with much greater control over the sound sources, indicate that the range

Loudness, Adaptation and Fatigue

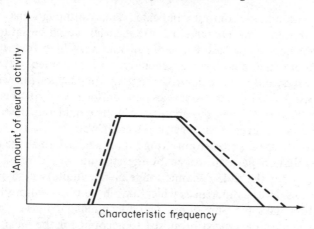

Figure 2.7 Idealised 'excitation pattern' for a tone at a high level. An increase in level, indicated by the dashed lines, produces no change in activity for the neurones in the centre of the pattern, since these are saturated. However, changes in neural activity do occur at the edge of the pattern. Note the greater growth of activity that occurs on the high-frequency side.

of thresholds for fibres with similar characteristic frequency is rather small. In the cat the range is about 20 dB (Kiang, 1968). Further, the individual fibres have a 'dynamic range' of only about 40 dB. In other words, an individual fibre will reach saturation firing rate within 40 dB of threshold (see Chapter 1, Figure 1.14). If changes in intensity were signalled as changes in firing rates of neurones with similar characteristic frequencies, then only a range of about 60 dB could be coded; for intensities greater than 60 dB above threshold all the neurones would be saturated (firing at their maximum rate). Clearly, then, we must seek some other mechanism for the coding of intensity changes at high intensities. One possibility lies in the way the 'excitation pattern' of the stimulus would spread with increasing intensity (see Figure 2.7). At high intensities neurones at the centre of the pattern would be saturated, but changes in intensity could be signalled by changes in the firing rate of neurones at the edge of the pattern.

It is not clear to what extent this argument could hold for the discrimination of wide-band stimuli, such as white noise. In theory the 'excitation pattern' for white noise has no edges, so that all fibres ought to be saturated by a noise of high intensity. However, we are not equally sensitive to all frequencies, as absolute threshold curves

69

and equal-loudness contours indicate. Thus, although the nerve fibres with mid-range characteristic frequencies would be saturated, this might not be the case for very low and very high frequencies. Furthermore, the stimuli have generally been presented via headphones which only pass a limited range of frequencies [in Miller's (1947) case the noise spectrum was only uniform (± 5 dB) between 150 and 7000 Hz]. Thus the acoustic stimuli would not have been truly wide-band, even if the electrical signals were.

We see, then, that changes in firing rate for neurones at the edges of the excitation pattern evoked by the stimulus could provide an explanation for the wide dynamic range of the auditory system. Let us now consider the differences which have been observed in the discrimination data for pure tones and for bursts of noise. Several different models have been proposed to account for the 'near miss' to Weber's Law for pure tones. Zwicker (1956, 1970), who worked with amplitude-modulated tones, suggested that a change in intensity can be detected whenever the 'excitation pattern' evoked by the stimulus changes somewhere by (about) 1 dB or more. At high levels the high-frequency side of the 'excitation pattern' grows more rapidly with increasing intensity than the rest of the pattern. This is deduced from changes in the shapes of masking patterns for tones in noise as a function of intensity (see Chapter 3). This non-linear growth in the 'excitation pattern' means that a 1 dB change in excitation on the high-frequency side will be produced by relatively smaller stimulus increments at high levels (see Figure 2.7). In support of this idea, Zwicker reported that the addition of a high-pass noise, which masks the high-frequency side of the excitation pattern but does not actually mask the tone, causes the DL for amplitude modulation at high intensities to approach that found at low levels.

McGill and Goldberg (1968a, b) presented an account of intensity discrimination based on neural counting mechanisms. They suggested that stimulus energies are 'mapped' into neural impulses whose number fluctuates from trial to trial even for non-varying stimuli. The number of neural impulses was assumed to follow a Poisson distribution. For this distribution the standard deviation equals the square root of the mean. If the mean number of neural impulses were proportional to stimulus energy (linear mapping), this would lead to a square root law for intensity discrimination ($\Delta I = k/I$, where k is a constant depending on the subject and the units used).

However, if the mapping follows a power law, as suggested by Stevens, then depending on the value of the exponent $(0 < \alpha < 1)$, a family of intensity discrimination functions is obtained which is bounded by Weber's Law on one side and the square root law on the other. An exponent of about 0.2 (so that the mean number of neural counts is proportional to $I^{0.2}$) produces a function which accords with the experimental data. Although this model is mathematically elegant, its assumptions about neural mapping are not well supported by physiological evidence. Further, the model does not take into account the spreading of the 'excitation pattern' which may be necessary to account for intensity discrimination at high levels.

A third explanation for the 'near miss' has been presented by Viemeister (1972), who suggested that the observers use information from aural harmonics. At high levels a single pure tone may produce in the ear a series of tones whose frequencies are multiples of the frequency of the tone which is physically presented. These tones, which are known as aural harmonics, behave like externally presented tones (e.g. they will 'beat' with a tone of slightly different frequency and they can be masked by bands of noise), and they probably arise as a result of some non-linear process in the middle or inner ear. Aural harmonics are negligible at low levels, but grow rapidly with intensity at high levels, so that a given change in stimulus level (in dB) may produce a somewhat larger change in level (in dB) of one or more of the aural harmonics. Thus, if observers can detect changes in the levels of the aural harmonics, their performance will improve at high levels. To test this explanation, Viemeister investigated the intensity discrimination of pulsed sinusoids, with a frequency of 950 Hz, in the presence of various types of filtered noise. He found little effect with a low-pass noise, whose cut-off frequency was 800 Hz, but a band-pass noise centred at the second aural harmonic ($f = 1900$ Hz) or a high-pass noise with cut-off at 1900 Hz both degraded performance at high levels. With the latter stimulus Weber's Law was obtained.

Moore and Raab (1974) provided a further test of Viemeister's model by using stimuli specifically designed to eliminate information from aural harmonics, namely tonal maskers with frequencies corresponding to those of the aural harmonics. These stimuli did affect discrimination, but only when they were at levels in excess of those which would be required to mask the aural harmonics. Masking stimuli at levels which were lower, but which should have been sufficiently intense to mask the aural harmonics (Clack, Erdreich and Knighton, 1972), had little effect on intensity discrimination, and did not eliminate the 'near miss'. Thus it seems likely that aural harmonics do not play an important role in intensity discrimination. This is confirmed by the results of Schacknow and Raab (1973) showing that the near miss is obtained for tone burst of frequency 7000 Hz. It seems extremely likely that aural harmonics could provide usable cues at such a high frequency.

In a second experiment Moore and Raab investigated the intensity discrimination of tone bursts ($f = 1000$ Hz) in the presence of three types of noise: wide-band, high-pass with cut-off frequency at 2000 Hz, and band-stop with cut-off frequencies at 500 Hz and 2000 Hz. Performance was unimpaired at low levels, but at high levels performance worsened, the greatest impairment being produced by the band-stop noise and the least by the wide-band noise. This experiment confirms that information at frequencies other than the nominal frequency of the test tone is important, but it further indicates that information on both the high- and low-frequency sides of the test tone affects intensity discrimination at high levels; the band-stop noise, which disrupts both types of information, had a greater effect than the high-pass noise, which only disrupts information on the high-frequency side.

It seems, then, that, at least for tones, information from the edges of the 'excitation pattern' allows improved performance at high levels. Some problems still remain, however. Firstly, we have to explain why information from the edges of the pattern allows improved performance for tones, but not for bands of noise. Secondly, we have to explain why performance is not *worse* at high levels than at low levels when the edges of the 'excitation pattern' are disrupted. For example, in the band-stop condition of Moore and Raab, the edges of the 'excitation pattern' on both the low- and high-frequency sides were disrupted, so that at the high level, where neurones at the centre of the pattern would have been saturated, performance should have been very poor. In fact, for this condition Weber's Law was found, so that performance was equally good at the high and low levels.

The answer to the first problem may be related to the stability of the edges of the 'excitation pattern'; a narrow band of noise will produce a pattern with edges, but the edges will be unstable because of the statistical properties of the noise. It may be that improved performance at high levels only occurs with stimuli which produce 'excitation patterns' with well-defined and stable edges. To answer the second problem it may be necessary to invoke some further mechanism for intensity discrimination. One possibility is that a regularity in the timing of neural impulses provides a cue as to the presence of a tone. When a tone is above threshold but is presented against a noise background, some neurones will be phase-locked to the tone, while neurones with characteristic frequencies far from that of the tone will show a quasi-random pattern of neural firing. When the tone is increased in intensity, more of the neurones will become phase-locked, and furthermore the degree of temporal regularity in the firing of neurones which are already phase-locked will increase, since the noise will now produce relatively less 'jitter'. Thus a change in temporal regularity of the patterns of neural firing will signal the intensity change of the tone. Such a mechanism would operate over a wide range of intensities, and would be little affected by saturation effects; temporal patterns of firing can alter even for neurones which are saturated. The mechanism would, however, be limited to frequencies below about 4–5 kHz.

It is possible that temporal patterns of neural firing contribute to the dynamic range of auditory neurones in another way. Hind (1972) has reported that 'we have commonly observed phase-locking at intensities below that required to raise the discharge rate above the spontaneous level'. Thus behavioural thresholds may be determined not by thresholds for increased firing in primary auditory neurones, but by thresholds for the detection of changes in temporal firing patterns. This would extend the effective dynamic range of single neurones. Note that, even for noise stimuli, the temporal patterns of firing are different from those for spontaneous activity (Ruggero, 1973). It is difficult to compare behavioural threshold with thresholds for increased firing rates in auditory neurones, since the methods of specifying stimulus level have not usually been comparable (cf. Elliot, Stein and Harrison, 1960; Kiang, 1968). There is a slight tendency for behavioural thresholds to be lower than 'neural' thresholds, but this discrepancy is also observed at high frequencies, where cues to phase-locking would not be available. Thus the role of temporal information in detecting at low levels must remain in doubt.

In some situations the wide dynamic range of the auditory system can be maintained even under conditions where cues to phase-locking would appear to be minimal. For example, Moore and Raab

(1975) investigated the intensity discrimination of a band of noise which was presented in the presence of a continuous band-stop background noise of sufficient intensity to disrupt information on both the high- and low-frequency sides of the excitation pattern evoked by the noise band. Performance did worsen slightly at high levels, but even at the highest levels used intensity discrimination was still quite good. Similar results have been reported by Viemeister (1974). Thus, even for a stimulus with little temporal regularity, such as a noise-band, neural saturation appears to have little effect on intensity discrimination.

Evans and Palmer (1975) have reported measurements on single neurones in the auditory nerve and cochlear nucleus of the cat, using stimulus presentations similar to those of Moore and Raab (1974, 1975) and Viemeister (1974). Firing rates of neurones were measured in response to changes in intensity of stimuli presented in band-stop background noises. As expected, the neurones in the auditory nerve did show saturation at high levels, but in the cochlear nucleus some neurones responded to signal-level changes in the presence of band-stop noise over a very wide intensity range, in many cases up to 100 dB above threshold. How the level signalling information is carried to the cochlear nucleus, by primary neurones which are presumably saturated, remains to be determined.

Recently it has been reported that not all primary auditory neurones show saturation within 40 dB of threshold (Sachs and Abbas, 1974). Instead the function relating rate of firing to stimulus level shows a bend at 20–30 dB above threshold, with rate continuing to increase gradually over another 30–40 dB. It may be that information from these units with 'sloping saturations' is sufficient to allow intensity discrimination at high levels. However, it is puzzling that performance does not worsen somewhat at high levels for a tone in band-stop noise, since the number of neurones signalling intensity changes should be considerably less at high levels than at low.

In summary, it seems likely that a number of different mechanisms play a role in intensity discrimination. For stimuli at low levels, intensity changes can be signalled both by changes in the firing rates of neurones at the centre of the 'excitation pattern', and by the spreading of the 'excitation pattern', so that more neurones are brought into operation. In addition, cues related to phase-locking may play a role in the detection of low-level tones. At high levels most of the neurones at the centre of the 'excitation pattern' may be saturated but intensity changes can still be signalled by the spread of the pattern and by changes in firing rate at the edges of the pattern. For stimuli producing 'excitation patterns' with stable edges, performance improves at high levels, and this may, in part, be related to a non-linear growth of excitation on the high-frequency side of the 'excitation pattern'. For periodic or quasi-periodic signals presented against noise backgrounds which disturb the edges of the 'excitation pattern', intensity changes may be signalled as changes in the degree of temporal regularity in the pattern of neural impulses. Alternatively, information from neurones with 'sloping saturations' may be sufficient to maintain performance at high levels.

Although this description of the mechanisms of intensity discrimination is plausible, it must still be considered as a preliminary framework in which to order the data, rather than a definitive and well-established theory. Furthermore, alternative ways of explaining the data, such as the neural counting mechanisms proposed by McGill and Goldberg (1968a, b), should be considered as complementary rather than opposing descriptions. It seems likely that statistical variability in the firing patterns of auditory neurones is responsible for the finite size of the intensity DL, and that the ultimate explanation of the intensity discrimination function observed for a given stimulus is to be sought in neural events. However, those neural events can only be defined by taking into account transformations of the stimulus in the auditory system.

2.7 LOUDNESS ADAPTATION, FATIGUE AND DAMAGE RISK

It is a property of all sensory systems that exposure to a stimulus of sufficient duration and intensity produces changes in the responsiveness of the system. Some changes occur during the presentation of the stimulus, so that its apparent magnitude decreases or it disappears completely (as sometimes happens for gustatory or olfactory stimuli). Other changes are apparent after the end of the stimulus; for example, shifts in threshold may occur. In general, such effects are much less marked in the auditory system than they are in, say, the visual system, although large threshold shifts are often observed after exposure to stimuli of very high intensity.

Hood (1950, 1972) has distinguished between auditory adaptation and auditory fatigue, and has emphasised that these are two quite distinct processes. The essential feature of fatigue is that it 'results from the application of a stimulus which is usually considerably in excess of that required to sustain the normal physiological response of the receptor, and it is measured after the stimulus has been removed' (Hood, 1972). For example, a subject's threshold at a particular frequency might be measured, after which the subject would be exposed to a fatiguing tone of a particular frequency and intensity for a period of time. The threshold would then be measured again, and the shift in threshold would be taken as a measure of fatigue. Notice that this procedure is concerned with 'the effect of an excessive stimulus upon a small and finite group of receptors, namely those which are normally brought into activity at near threshold intensities'. Auditory fatigue defined in this way is more properly referred to as post-stimulatory auditory fatigue, and the measure used is called temporary threshold shift (TTS).

Auditory adaptation has as its essential feature the process of 'equilibration'. The response of a receptor to a steady stimulus declines as a function of time until it reaches a steady level at which the energy expended by the receptor is just balanced by the metabolic energy which becomes available to sustain it. The psychological counterpart of this is a decline in the apparent magnitude of a stimulus (e.g. its loudness) during the first few minutes of presentation, followed by a period in which the apparent magnitude remains roughly constant. Auditory adaptation can be studied by means of loudness balance tests. For example, a tone of fixed intensity, say 80 dB SPL, is applied to the subject's left or test ear, and a loudness balance is made with a tone of the same frequency but variable level applied to the right or control ear. For a normal subject this balance will be obtained with an intensity of about 80 dB SPL. The tone in the right ear is now removed, but that in the left is continued for a further 3 min. Following this adaptation period, a loudness balance is established once again, and it is generally found that the tone in the right ear now produces a loudness match at a lower level, say 60 dB SPL. Thus the amount of adaptation corresponds to an intensity change of 20 dB. Notice that the measurement of the decrement of response takes place while the adapting stimulus is being applied.

There are several problems associated with this technique of simultaneous dichotic loudness balance (SDLB). Firstly, adaptation may occur in the control ear, either by means of central neural effects, or by physical cross-over of the sound, which occurs at 40–50 dB SL in the frequency range from 100 to 10 000 Hz (von Békésy and Rosenblith, 1951). Secondly, if the control tone is presented continuously during a loudness balance, this, too, may introduce adaptation in the control ear. Various other factors, such as the specific method of presentation, have also been shown to affect the results. Finally, it is not clear whether the balance is made on the basis of loudness *per se*, or on the basis of the lateralised image within the head.

Recently a number of papers have appeared which indicate that if the test conditions are designed to eliminate lateralising effects and binaural interaction between adapting and comparison tones, then suprathreshold loudness adaptation is essentially absent (e.g. Bray, Dirks and Morgan, 1973). One technique makes use of a comparison tone whose frequency differs from that of the adapting tone. The adapting tone is presented continuously to one ear, while the comparison tone is presented intermittently to the other. This technique is called a simultaneous heterophonic-loudness balance technique (the corresponding name for the case when adapting and comparison tones have the same frequency is homophonic). An alternative is to use a monaural heterophonic technique, where adapting and comparison tones are presented to the same ear, but are sufficiently different in frequency (say 500 Hz and 10 000 Hz) for adaptation to one to have little effect on the loudness of the other. A third technique requires the subject to adjust the intensity of a continuously presented sound so as to maintain it at constant loudness. If the subject increases the intensity of the sound with increasing duration of presentation, then this indicates that adaptation is occurring. Most of the workers using these techniques have reported that there is no significant loudness adaptation for adapting tones between 50 and 90 dB SPL. This has been taken to indicate that the effects which are observed for the homophonic SDLB test are mediated by central interactions, and should not be interpreted as indicating a genuine decrement in loudness for a continuously presented stimulus. On the other hand, there is at least one report (Weiler and Friedman, 1973) of significant (greater than 20 dB) adaptation obtained using a monaural heterophonic technique, so that not all adaptation phenomena can be attributed to binaural interactions. At the present time no clear reasons can be given for the differences between the different methods, and the results presented later should be treated with caution until such reasons are forthcoming.

Although there is a great deal of evidence that fatigue and adaptation are distinct phenomena, at both the physiological and psychological level, they are not always easy to distinguish. As Elliot and Fraser (1970) have pointed out, '. . . the question continues to plague investigators as to whether, when the ear is stimulated, for example with a 60– or 80–dB tone, the changes observed during stimulation, or immediately after its cessation are primarily indicative of adaptation or of fatigue. Consequently, although the terms are well established, we are using them with the realization that they often do not refer to completely independent physiological processes.'

We will not attempt here to give a detailed account of the physiological processes involved in fatigue and adaptation, or of the factors which affect these. For a review of these the reader is referred to Elliot and Fraser (1970). They conclude that '. . . stimulation results in reversible neural changes that indicate neural adaptation, reduction in hair-cell response, and in all probability, a variety of cochlear environmental changes that interfere with both hair-cell and nerve-cell functioning'. In very general terms, the properties of adaptation (as defined by loudness balance tests) seem to parallel those of neural adaptation, while fatigue seems to be connected with hair cell changes.

2.7.1 *Post-stimulatory auditory fatigue*

The most common index of auditory fatigue is the TTS, whose measurement was described briefly above. One problem with measuring the TTS is that the recovery process may be quite rapid, so that a threshold measurement has to be obtained as quickly as possible; but this in turn can lead to inaccuracies in the measurement. The most common method is to use a motor-driven attenuator, which the subject controls so as to maintain the level of the tone as close as possible to threshold. Sometimes continuous tones are used, but since subjects often have difficulty in tracking these, pulsed tones are generally preferred.

There are five major factors which influence the size of the TTS: (1) the time between cessation of the fatiguing stimulus and the post-exposure threshold determination—called the recovery interval (RI); (2) the intensity of the fatiguing stimulus (I); (3) the duration of the fatiguing stimulus (D); (4) the frequency of the fatiguing stimulus (F_e); and (5) the frequency of the test stimulus (F_t). We will briefly summarise the effects of each of these.

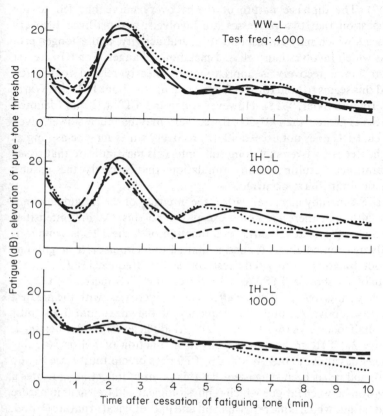

Figure 2.8   Recovery curves illustrating the elevation in threshold produced by a fatiguing tone of 500 Hz at 120 dB SPL for 3 min. Test tones of 4 kHz (two subjects) and 1 kHz (one subject) were used, and each set of curves represents retests under identical conditions. Note the 'bounce' that occurs at 2 min for the 4 kHz test tones. From Hirsh and Ward (1952), by permission of the authors and the *Journal of the Acoustical Society of America.*

TTS generally becomes smaller the longer RI, although for many conditions the recovery curve is diphasic; recovery from the large TTS immediately following exposure is often followed by a 'bounce', particularly at high frequencies. Thus a valley at RI = 1 min is often followed by a bounce at RI = 2 min (see Figure 2.8). Sometimes the initial recovery process may actually overshoot the original threshold level, so that a temporary sensitisation occurs (Hughes and Rosenblith,

1957). The diphasic nature of the recovery curve has led to the suggestion that two processes are involved; a short-lived recovery process which may correspond to neural activity, and a longer process which involves hair cell and metabolic changes. For RIs greater than 2 min, recovery is approximately linearly related to log RI, and this seems to hold for RIs from 2 min up to about 112 min (Ward, Glorig and Sklar, 1958). However, when the TTS at 2 min (denoted TTS_2) is greater than 40–50 dB, recovery may be much slower. Even when TTS_2 does not exceed 40 dB, recovery times may be as long as 16 h. Recovery over such long time intervals may indicate that tissue alterations, resulting from stimulation that exceeds the tissue's elastic limits, have occurred.

TTS generally increases with I, the intensity of the fatiguing stimulus, although there are some exceptions to this. At low intensities TTS changes relatively little as a function of I, the TTS is symmetrically distributed about F_e, and is limited to its immediate neighbourhood. In other words, only test tones with frequencies F_t close to that of F_e show a TTS. As I increases, the TTS increases, the frequency range over which the effects occur increases, with the greatest increase above F_e, and the frequency of the maximum TTS shifts one-half octave or more above F_e. At high levels, and when F_t is above F_e, TTS grows very rapidly as a function of I. For fatiguing intensities above about 90–100 dB, TTS rises precipitously (see Figure 2.9), and it has been suggested that this point of inflection indicates a division between fatigue which is physiological and transient in nature and fatigue which is more permanent and pathological in nature (Hood, 1950; Hirsh and Bilger, 1955). The upward frequency shift in F_t at which the maximum TTS occurs is not fully understood, but it may be related to the mechanical properties of the basilar membrane. The non-linearity observed by Rhode (1971) is consistent with shifts in the vibration envelope towards the basal (high-frequency) end of the basilar membrane with increasing amplitude of a sinusoidal stimulus.

Fatigue generally increases with duration, and a number of workers have reported that TTS is linearly related to log D (Hood, 1950; Ward *et al.*, 1958). However, for low frequencies, particularly when the fatiguing stimulus is noise or a rapidly interrupted tone (Ward, 1963), the growth rate is reduced, probably because the aural reflex (a contraction of the middle-ear muscles in response to intense sounds) reduces sound transmission. The log D function probably also does not extend below a D of 5 min.

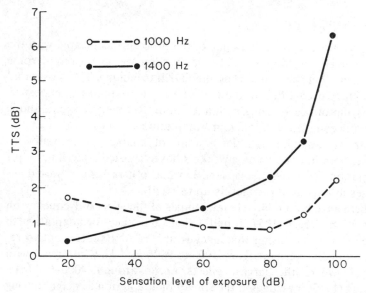

Figure 2.9 Increases in TTS with increases in the level of the 1 kHz fatiguing tone. Test tones of 1 kHz and 1.4 kHz were used. Note that for high exposure levels the function accelerates, and that the TTS is greater for a frequency above that of the fatiguing tone than for a tone at that frequency. From Hirsh and Bilger (1955), by permission of the authors and the *Journal of the Acoustical Society of America*.

Fatigue effects are generally more marked at high frequencies, at least up to 4–6 kHz. Thus when the fatiguing stimulus is a broadband noise, maximum TTSs occur between 4 and 6 kHz. It is also the case that permanent hearing losses, resulting from the exposure to intense sounds, or from old age, tend to be greatest in this region. Both of these may result from the greater stiffness of the high-frequency portions of the basilar membrane, so that elastic limits are more easily exceeded.

Recently a number of studies have appeared reporting the effects of exposure to environmental noise of various kinds, including rock and roll music. Harris (1972) in a review of these concluded that '. . . the quieter bands may be harmless, but if the amplification/reverberation condition reaches 110 dBA, a sizeable fraction of persons would be adversely affected probably permanently; while a 120 dBA level, at which some music groups have registered, would create havoc with most audiograms'.

2.7.2 *Auditory adaptation*

We have already discussed some of the problems associated with the measurement of adaptation. In this section we shall present some general findings obtained using the SDLB technique. The most rapid adaptation occurs during the first one or two minutes of exposure, the asymptotic level being within 3–7 min. Recovery is rapid, and is generally complete within 2 min. Adaptation occurs at both high and low intensities, although the amount of adaptation generally increases with intensity. Some workers have reported a levelling off of adaptation for levels above 60 dB, while others have reported increases in adaptation for levels up to 80 dB.

There have been relatively few studies of the effect of frequency on adaptation. Jerger (1957) found a slight tendency for adaptation to increase with increasing frequency from 125 to 1000 Hz, but to remain roughly constant from 1000 to 8000 Hz. This contrasts with fatigue, where the largest effects occur around 4000–6000 Hz. Thwing (1955) investigated the spread of adaptation to neighbouring frequencies for a 1000 Hz tone at 80 db SPL, and found a maximum effect at the adapting frequency, with continuously decreasing effects for frequencies on either side. He suggested that the adaptation is proportional to the extent to which excitation pattern of the comparison and adapting stimulus overlap. More data are needed for the evaluation of this hypothesis.

2.8 LOUDNESS RECRUITMENT, ADAPTATION AND FATIGUE IN THE ASSESSMENT OF DEAFNESS

Hearing losses may be broadly categorised into two main types. The first type, conductive deafness, occurs when there is some defect, usually in the middle ear, which reduces the transmission of sound to the inner ear. For example, a growth may occur on the eardrum, or the bones in the middle ear may ossify or stick together. In general, this results in a more or less uniform hearing loss as a function of frequency, and the difficulty experienced by the sufferer can be well predicted from his threshold elevation. A simple hearing aid is usually quite effective in such cases.

The second type of hearing loss is called nerve deafness, or sensorineural hearing loss. In general, the extent of the loss increases with frequency, but the difficulty experienced by the sufferer may not be well predicted from the audiogram. Sensorineural hearing loss may arise as a result of defects in many different parts of the auditory system, and the particular difficulties experienced by the sufferer, and the types of symptoms exhibited, depend on which part of the system is affected. Patients often have difficulty in understanding speech in noisy environments, and the condition is usually not completely alleviated by a hearing aid.

2.8.1 *Recruitment*

One phenomenon which often occurs when there are lesions of the cochlea itself is loudness recruitment. This refers to an unusually rapid growth of loudness as the Sensation Level of a tone is increased, and it might be observed as follows. Suppose that a patient has a hearing loss at 4000 Hz of 60 dB in one ear only. If a 4000 Hz tone is introduced into his normal ear at 100 dB SPL (which would also be about 100 dB above threshold for that ear), then the tone which sounds equally loud in his poor ear will also be about 100 dB SPL. Thus a tone which is only 40 dB above threshold in his poor ear may sound as loud as a tone which is 100 dB above threshold in his good ear; the ear with recruitment seems to 'catch up' with the normal ear in loudness. Notice that although recruitment is normally regarded as pathological, a phenomenon very much like it occurs in normal listeners for tones of very high and very low frequency. The loudness of these tones grows more rapidly per decibel than does the loudness for tones of middle frequencies.

There are a number of different ways of measuring or detecting recruitment. One indirect way is to measure the difference limen (DL) for intensity. The reasoning behind this is as follows: if loudness is increasing more rapidly than normal as the stimulus intensity is increased, a smaller than normal intensity change will be required for a just noticeable difference in loudness (in fact this does not follow logically, since the size of the DL is limited by variability in the loudness sensation, as well as its rate of growth). In general, recruitment is most marked at low sensation levels, so that if this reasoning is correct, the DL should be abnormally small at low sensation levels but should approach the normal DL at high levels, where the rate of growth of loudness is more nearly normal. This, in fact, turns out to be the case. For normal subjects the intensity DL at low sensation levels is larger than that at higher levels, whereas for patients with recruitment the DL remains constant or decreases at very low levels, depending on the amount of recruitment.

A second technique for measuring recruitment is the alternate binaural loudness balance (ABLB) test, which can be applied when only one ear is affected. A tone of a given intensity at the good ear is alternated with a variable tone, of the same frequency, at the affected ear, and a loudness match is obtained. This is repeated at a number of different intensities, so that the rate of growth of loudness in the affected ear can be compared with that in the good ear. Hood (1972) has emphasised the importance of presenting the tones alternately at the two ears, rather than presenting sustained tones simultaneously at the two ears. The reason for this is that recruitment is essentially a function of the on-effect, the initial response to a stimulus; for sustained tones pathological adaptation (see below) may occur, so that the loudness decreases rapidly with increasing duration of the stimulus. Thus all tests designed to detect recruitment must involve either interrupted tones or abrupt changes in tonal intensity. A third test for recruitment involves the measurement of Loudness Discomfort Levels (LDLs). For most normal subjects a tone becomes uncomfortably loud when its level reaches 100–110 dB SPL. For a patient with a non-recruiting hearing loss the LDL may be much higher, whereas, if recruitment is present, the LDL will fall within the range for normal subjects. The phenomenon of recruitment probably accounts for a statement which is often heard from patients with this type of hearing loss: 'Don't shout; you're talking loud enough, but I can't understand what you are saying!' The patient may not be able to hear very faint sounds, but sounds of high intensity are just as loud to him as to a normal listener. However, sounds which are easily audible may not be easily intelligible.

The physiological causes of recruitment are not entirely clear, but it occurs consistently in lesions of the cochlea, and is usually absent in conductive deafness and in retrocochlear deafness (deafness due to neural disturbances occurring at a higher point in the auditory pathway than the cochlea). It is probably connected with hair cell damage, and in particular with damage to the outer hair cells. If the responses of auditory nerve fibres to low level stimuli are determined primarily by input from the outer hair cells, then a loss of these hair cells would lead to an elevation in threshold. If, however, the response at high levels is determined primarily by input from the inner hair cells, and if these are normal, then response patterns at high levels will be normal. Thus the sensation of loudness at high levels will be normal, even though thresholds are elevated. Measurements of the cochlear microphonic response have indicated functional differences between inner and outer hair cells. Karlan, Tonndorf and Khanna (1972) have suggested that the two sets of generators (inner and outer hair cells) have different thresholds and different gains (rate of change of output as a function of the intensity of the stimulus), while Dallos *et al.* (1972) have suggested that potentials produced by inner hair cells are proportional to the velocity of the basilar membrane, and potentials generated by outer hair cells are proportional to the displacement of the basilar membrane. It is certainly the case that the outer hair cells are the most susceptible to damage (e.g. from intense auditory stimulation), and the anatomical evidence is consistent with the idea that it is the disproportion between the numbers of inner and outer hair cells that provides the basis for many types of loudness recruitment (Schuknecht, 1970). However, there have been reports (Dix and Hood, 1973) of recruitment caused by brain-stem disorders.

2.8.2 *Pathological adaptation*

Abnormal metabolic processes in the cochlea or auditory nerve sometimes result in a very rapid decrease in neural responses, although the on-effect may be normal or near-normal. The psychological correlate of this is adaptation, which is more extreme and more rapid than normal. It turns out to be the case that this effect is usually greater in lesions of the nerve fibres than of the cochlea itself, and so pathological adaptation is useful in the differential diagnosis of cochlear and retrocochlear lesions. There are several ways of studying this phenomenon, including the simultaneous dichotic loudness balance procedure which we described for normal adaptation. Since, however, pathological adaptation occurs at all intensity levels, it can be conveniently studied with tones close to threshold. One way of doing this is to measure the difference in threshold for continuous and interrupted tones. For patients with conductive deafness, or for normal subjects, there is little difference between the two types of theshold. For a patient with retrocochlear lesions the threshold for a continuous tone may be considerably higher than that for an interrupted tone. One very striking way of demonstrating this is to first determine the threshold for an interrupted tone. The intensity is then raised by 5 dB and the tone is presented continuously. After five or six seconds the sensation of tone will disappear completely, although for the normal listener the sensation would persist indefinitely. It is often necessary to raise the intensity of the tone by 20–30 dB before the sensation persists indefinitely for the subject with retrocochlear lesions. It is easy to confirm that the effect is pathological adaptation rather than fatigue, by interrupting the tone at any time during the test; the original threshold is restored at once. These tests are known as tone-decay tests.

It is clear that measures of recruitment and adaptation are of considerable use in the diagnosis of hearing disorders, and in the separation of different types of hearing loss. Such measures also give us a valuable insight into the relationship between normal and abnormal functioning of the auditory system, and thus provide pointers for the direction of research in these areas. Studies of what can go wrong with the auditory system help us to understand how it normally works, and conversely a more complete knowledge of how the normal system functions is essential if we are to be able to work out exactly what has gone wrong in cases of hearing loss. A knowledge of underlying processes involved in adaptation and fatigue is important in the interpretation of clinical data, and also indicates the need, as Hood (1972) puts it '. . . for care in the design and execution of all audiological test procedures'.

2.9 GENERAL CONCLUSIONS

In this chapter we have discussed a number of different aspects of the perception of loudness and the way it is coded in the auditory system. Absolute threshold curves show that we are most sensitive to middle frequencies, at least part of this sensitivity arising from the action of the middle ear. Our absolute sensitivity is such that our ability to detect faint sounds would normally be limited by environmental noises, rather than by limits in the system itself. There is, however, considerable variability between different individuals, so that thresholds 20 dB on either side of the mean are still considered as 'normal'. Hearing losses with age are most marked at high frequencies, but unless some pathological condition occurs, the reception of frequencies important for speech perception deteriorates very little with age.

Equal-loudness contours allow us to compare the loudnesses of sounds of different frequencies. In general, the shapes of equal-loudness contours are similar to absolute threshold curves at low levels, but become flatter at high levels. Thus at high levels it is roughly true that tones of equal SPL sound equally loud regardless of frequency. The shapes of equal-loudness contours indicate that loudness grows more rapidly for low frequencies and for very high frequencies than for middle frequencies. This means that the tonal balance of recorded sounds, such as speech or music, may be affected by the level at which the sounds are reproduced. Equal-loudness contours are used in the design of sound level meters, so that the readings obtained give a better indication of the perceived loudness than would readings based simply on physical intensity.

The technique of magnitude estimation allows the construction of 'psychological' scales of loudness, the most common one being the sone scale suggested by S. S. Stevens. Such scales give a set of numbers which relate the perceived loudness of a given sound to its physical characteristics (such as intensity), and they have been utilised in models which allow the calculation of the loudness of any complex sound. The validity of such scales has been questioned, however, and at present there seems to be no well-established and generally accepted method for calculating loudness.

Absolute intensive thresholds, masked thresholds and the loudness of sounds all depend upon duration. Over a certain range of durations (about 15–150 ms) the ear appears to integrate sound energy for the purpose of detection. Thus it is approximately true that threshold depends only on the total amount of energy in the stimulus, and not on how that energy is distributed over time. However, this does not hold at very long durations, probably because of the limited 'integration time' of the ear. At very short durations 'energy splatter' in the signal may also reduce its detectability. There is some evidence that the 'integration time' of the ear is shorter for high frequencies than for low. The loudness of short-duration sounds may also depend upon their total energy, but the results are much less clear-cut, and vary considerably according to the experimental technique used.

We are able to detect changes in intensity for a wide range of intensities and for many types of stimuli. In general, discrimination performance, as measured by the Weber fraction ($\Delta I/I$), is independent of level for bands of noise, but improves at high levels for pure tones. Various psychoacoustic experiments indicate that at high levels information at frequencies above and (to a lesser extent) below the frequency of the test tone may be important in intensity discrimination. These results, together with the neurophysiological data, indicate that a number of different sources of sensory information may be used in detecting intensity changes. These include the spreading of the excitation pattern with increasing level, the non-linear growth of the excitation pattern on the high-frequency side, and for periodic stimuli the regularities in the temporal patterns of neural firing.

Exposure to auditory stimulation produces two types of changes in the responsiveness of the system: the apparent magnitude of the stimulus may decrease, a process known as adaptation, and the absolute threshold measured after the offset of the stimulus may be elevated, a process known as fatigue. There are many problems associated with the measurement of these processes, and they are not always clearly separable. However, the properties of adaptation seem to parallel those of neural adaptation, while fatigue seems to be connected with hair cell changes.

Fatigue, or temporary threshold shift (TTS), generally decreases with increasing recovery time, although a 'bounce' sometimes occurs about two minutes after cessation of the fatiguing stimulus. This may indicate that more than one process is involved in recovery. Recovery times vary considerably, but may be as long as 16 h or more. TTS is generally small at low intensities, but increases rapidly when the fatiguing stimulus is above about 90–100 dB SPL. This may indicate a division between fatigue which is physiological and transient in nature and fatigue which is more permanent and pathological in nature. Sound levels above 110–120 dB SPL may produce permanent hearing losses, particularly if exposure is of long duration. Such sound levels have been registered by some music groups, and also may be easily attained by many of the sets of headphones which are available on the domestic market.

Adaptation effects measured using the SDLB technique are generally quite rapid, the greatest adaptation occurring within one or two minutes of exposure. Recovery is also rapid. Adaptation occurs at both high and low levels, but is greatest at high levels. Some workers have reported a levelling off of adaptation for levels above 60 dB, while others have reported increases for levels up to 80 dB. A number of recent studies using methods which avoid binaural interaction have indicated that loudness adaptation is essentially absent in normal ears at moderate intensities. The reasons for the discrepancies between different methods remain to be explained.

In some cases of deafness, particularly when there is pathology of cochlea itself, loudness recruitment may occur. Recruitment is an abnormally rapid growth of loudness with increase in intensity: the sufferer may have an elevated threshold, but intense sounds are as loud to him as to a normal listener. The phenomenon may be detected in a variety of ways, either indirectly by the measurement of an abnormally small intensity difference limen at low sensation levels or, when only one ear is affected, by direct comparison with the good ear, using a loudness balancing technique. Recruitment may be connected with hair cell damage and, in particular, with a disproportion between the numbers of inner and outer hair cell.

Pathological adaptation may occur when there are abnormal metabolic processes in the cochlea or auditory nerve, although the effect is usually greater in the latter case. The adaptation is more rapid and more extreme than normal, and is most easily measured for tones close to threshold; a continuous tone just above threshold may fade after a time and eventually become completely inaudible. However, the tone may easily be made audible once again by interrupting it.

Recruitment and pathological adaptation are useful measures in the differential diagnosis of cochlear and retrocochlear lesions, and in addition they provide useful insights into the functioning of the auditory system. It is to be hoped that the future will see an increasing co-operation between clinical audiologists and otologists and the basic scientist. Theories about normal auditory functioning cannot be complete if they do not take into account the phenomena (such as recruitment) which are observed clinically, and clinical workers have much to gain from theories and data derived from studies of the normal human subject.

3

Frequency Analysis, Masking and the Critical Band

3.1 INTRODUCTION

It is a matter of everyday experience that one sound may be obscured, or rendered inaudible, in the presence of other sounds. Thus music from a car radio may mask the sound of the car's engine, provided that the music is somewhat more intense. Masking has been defined as: '(1) The *process* by which the threshold of audibility for one sound is raised by the presence of another (masking) sound. (2) The *amount* by which the threshold of audibility of a sound is raised by the presence of another (masking) sound. The unit customarily used is the decibel.' (American Standards Association, 1960.)

It is perhaps unfortunate that this definition includes the observed masking effect as well as the underlying masking processes. Further, the definition does not take into account the phenomenon of partial masking (Scharf, 1971), whereby the loudness of a sound may be decreased by another sound without actually becoming completely inaudible. For the moment, however, we will continue to use the A.S.A. definition.

Hearing theorists have for many years been interested in the physical parameters which affect the masking of one sound by another. The experimental results can tell us a great deal about how the auditory system analyses and discriminates the various components in a mixture of sounds, and the limits of this analysing faculty may allow us to make certain inferences about the processes involved in masking. In addition, a knowledge of the rules governing the masking of one sound by another can be very useful in practical situations. For example, one might want to know the extent to which noise from new machinery in a factory will interfere with the ability of workers to hold conversations or to detect warning signals. One very general result which arose from the early experiments was that a signal will most easily be masked by a sound having frequency components close to, or the same as, those of the signal. This led to the idea that our ability to separate out the elements of a complex sound depends, at least in part, on the frequency-resolving power of the basilar membrane. Fletcher, in 1940, formalised this idea with the concept of the critical band (see below). A different kind of masking, called central masking, has been described by Zwislocki (1971). In central masking the threshold of a signal presented to one ear is elevated by a masking sound presented to the other ear. The name 'central' is used because this masking cannot be ascribed to processes in the ear itself (i.e. peripheral processes) but must arise at or beyond the point in the auditory system where inputs from the two ears are combined (i.e. centrally). The threshold shift in central masking is generally small, and rarely exceeds 10 dB.

A second important physical parameter which affects masking is time. Most of this chapter will be devoted to simultaneous masking, in which the signal is presented at the same time as the masker. Later on we will discuss forward masking, in which a signal is masked by a preceding masker, and backward masking, in which the masker follows a signal.

3.2   THE CRITICAL BAND CONCEPT

Wegel and Lane (1924) published the first systematic investigation of the masking of one pure tone by another. They determined the threshold of audibility of a tone with adjustable frequency in the presence of a masker with fixed frequency and intensity. The graph plotting masked threshold as a function of the frequency of the adjustable tone is known as a masked audiogram. The results of Wegel and Lane were complicated by the occurrence of beats when the signal and masker were close together in frequency. Beats occur because of the changing phase relationship between the signal and masker, which causes the two sounds alternately to reinforce and cancel one another. The resulting amplitude fluctuations occur at a rate equal to the frequency difference between the two tones, and if this rate is not too rapid, audible loudness fluctuations occur. Beats can provide a cue to the presence of the signal even if the signal itself is not audible, and to avoid this problem later experimenters (for

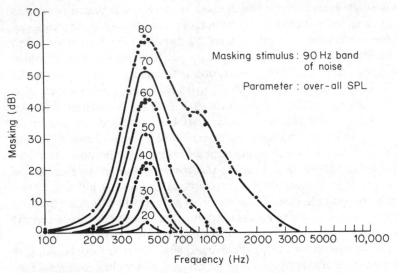

Figure 3.1 Masked audiograms for a narrow band of noise centred at 410 Hz. Each curve shows the elevation in pure-tone threshold as a function of frequency for a particular level of the masking noise. From Egan and Hake (1950), by permission of the authors and the *Journal of the Acoustical Society of America.*

example, Greenwood, 1961) have used a narrow band of noise as either the signal or masker. Such a noise has 'built in' amplitude fluctuations, and in addition does not produce regular beats when added to a tone.

The masked threshold curves obtained in these experiments show steep slopes on the low-frequency side, of between 80 and 240 dB/octave for pure-tone masking, and 55–190 dB/octave for narrowband noise masking. The slopes on the high-frequency side are less steep and depend to some extent on the level of the masker. A typical set of results is shown in Figure 3.1. Notice that on the high-frequency side the slopes of the curves tend to become shallower at high levels. Thus if the level of a low-frequency masker is increased by, say, 10 dB, the masked threshold of a high-frequency signal may be elevated by more than 10 dB; the amount of masking grows nonlinearly on the high-frequency side. This result has certain practical implications for the reproduction of sounds such as speech. Each frequency component in a speech sound will have a masking effect on adjacent frequency components. As the overall level is increased, the low frequencies become more and more effective in masking the higher ones, so that ultimately this 'upward spread of masking' results in a loss of audibility of the important information-carrying mid- to high-frequency components. The result is that reproduced speech is less intelligible at high overall listening levels. Overall these results confirm Mayer's (1894) observation that it is easier to mask a tone by a second tone of lower frequency than by one of higher frequency, and that frequencies near the signal are more effective than frequencies farther removed.

Fletcher (1940) attempted to account for these results, and for many of the other phenomena of masking, with the *critical band* concept. He suggested that different frequencies produce their maximal effects at different locations along the basilar membrane, so that each location responds only to a limited range of frequencies. The effective frequency range to which a given location (or filter) responds is its critical band. According to Fletcher, masking will occur whenever a masking sound produces a maximum rate of neural discharge in a channel (derived from one filter or critical band) which would otherwise respond to the signal.

Fletcher suggested that the critical band could be determined by measuring the masked threshold of a tone in broad-band white noise, given the following hypotheses.

(1) Only a narrow band of frequencies surrounding the tone—the critical band—contribute to the masking of the tone.

(2) When the noise just masks the tone, the power of the noise inside the critical band is equal to the power of the tone. Noise power is usually specified in terms of the power in a band of frequencies 1 Hz wide (say from 1000 Hz to 1001 Hz). This is called the noise power density, and is denoted by the symbol N_0. For a white noise N_0 is independent of frequency, so that the total noise power in a band of frequencies W Hz wide is $N_0 \times W$. According to Fletcher, when this width equals the critical bandwidth, the total power in the band will equal the power, P, of the tone at threshold. Thus W is equal to P/N_0, and by measuring P and N_0 we can evaluate W.

The first hypothesis has been confirmed by experiments in which the threshold of a tone is measured in noise of various bandwidths

(Hamilton, 1957; Greenwood, 1961). Increases in noise bandwidth beyond a certain critical value have little effect on the threshold of a tone. However, the second hypothesis has turned out not to be strictly accurate (Scharf, 1970); at most frequencies this hypothesis leads to estimates of the critical bandwidth which are about two and one-half times smaller than estimates obtained by more direct methods (see below). For this reason the values obtained by Fletcher's method (see, for example, Hawkins and Stevens, 1950) are called critical ratios, and the term 'critical bandwidth' is reserved for more direct measurements of the bandwidth of a complex stimuli or of maskers at which the pattern of responses obtained in various psychoacoustical tasks changes rather abruptly. The difference between the critical ratio function and the generally accepted critical band function is illustrated in Figure 3.2.

The discussion so far may have led the reader to believe that the critical band behaves like a perfect rectangular filter, so that sounds whose frequencies are separated by more than a critical band will not interact in any way. This, in fact, is not the case, since, for example, one tone may mask another over frequency separations considerably greater than a critical band. We are led, then, to consider the critical band as resembling a filter with sloping edges; the actual critical bandwidth is some measure of the 'effective' bandwidth of this filter. Swets, Green and Tanner (1962) have shown, using the theory of signal detectability (see Section 3.7) that estimates of the critical bandwidth derived from masking experiments may vary according to the assumed filter shape. Just what this shape ought to be is not, at the present time, clear, although ways of approaching this problem are now being developed (Patterson, 1974, 1976).

Another question which arises is whether there is only a discrete number of critical bands, each one adjacent to its neighbours, or whether there is a continuous series of overlapping critical bands. For convenience, data relating to critical bands have often been presented as though the former were the case. For example, Scharf (1970) presented a table showing critical bandwidths for 24 successive critical bands, the upper cut-off frequency for each band being the same as the lower cut-off for the next highest band. While this method of presentation is convenient, it seems clear that critical bands are continuous rather than discrete; there has been no experimental evidence for any discontinuity or break between different

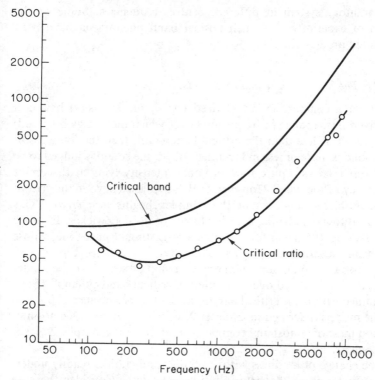

Figure 3.2 A comparison of the width, Δf, of the critical band as determined by direct measures and as determined from the critical ratio. From Zwicker *et al.* (1957), by permission of the authors and the *Journal of the Acoustical Society of America.*

critical bands. Thus we may talk about the critical band around any frequency in the audible range which we care to choose.

Since Fletcher first described the critical band concept, a large number of different types of experiment have shown that listeners' responses to complex sounds differ according to whether the stimuli are wider or narrower than the critical band. Further, these different experiments give remarkably similar estimates both of the absolute width of the critical band and of the way the critical band varies as a function of frequency. Thus the critical band phenomenon pervades and summarises a great variety of data, and provides a valuable guide in the planning of experiments and the analysis of data. For example, it may be used as an indication of the spectral resolution of the auditory system at different centre frequencies. Some of the types of experiment in which critical band phenomena have been observed are described below.

3.2.1 *The loudness of complex sounds*

Consider a complex sound of fixed energy (or intensity) having a bandwidth (the range of frequencies over which the energy is spread) of *W*. If *W* is less than the critical bandwidth, then the loudness of the sound is more or less independent of *W*; the sound is judged to be about as loud as a pure tone of equal intensity lying at the centre frequency of the band. However, if *W* is increased beyond the critical bandwidth, the loudness of the complex begins to *increase*. This has been found to be the case for bands of noise (Zwicker, Flottorp and Stevens, 1957) and for complexes consisting of pure tones whose frequency separation is varied (Sharf, 1961, 1970) (see Figure 3.3). Thus, for a given amount of energy, a complex sound will be louder if the energy is spread over a number of critical bands, than if it is all contained within one critical band. This finding has been incorporated in the models described in Chapter 2, which allow the calculation of the loudness of almost any complex sound (see, for example, Zwicker and Scharf, 1965).

The change of loudness with stimulus bandwidth is readily understood in terms of the neurophysiological data. Consider the case where two tones, close together in frequency, are presented. The two tones will fall within the same critical band, and to a large extent will excite the same set of neurones. Now at moderate and high intensities the firing rates of individual neurones change relatively slowly as a function of intensity, so that the total number of neural firings in response to the two tones will not be much greater than the number which would occur in response to either tone alone. If, on the other hand, the two tones are widely separated in frequency, so that they fall in different critical bands, they will excite essentially independent sets of neurones. The total number of neural impulses will then be roughly double that which would occur in response to either tone presented alone. If, then, loudness is at least related to the total number of neural impulses evoked by the stimulus, it is clear that the loudness of the complex will be greater when the components fall in different critical bands than when they fall in the same critical band. The argument can easily be extended to cover multiple-com-

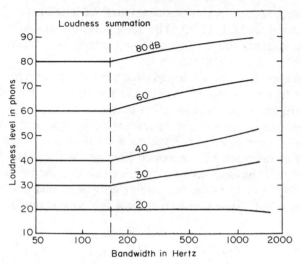

Figure 3.3 The loudness level in phons of a band of noise centred at 1 kHz, measured as a function of the width of the band. For each of the curves the overall SPL is constant and is indicated in the figure. The dashed line shows that the bandwidth at which loudness begins to increase is the same at all levels tested (except that no increase occurs at the lowest level). From Feldtkeller and Zwicker (1956), by permission of the authors and publisher.

ponent complex tones, and bands of noise. Another factor which might affect the number of neural firings evoked by a complex stimulus is the lateral suppression which has been observed on the basilar membrane (Rhode and Robles, 1974) and in auditory nerve fibres (see Chapter 1). This lateral suppression would reduce the total number of neural firings evoked by a complex stimulus when the components were within a certain frequency range, but would have little effect when components were widely spaced in frequency. Thus the critical band may also reflect the effective frequency range over which the suppression effects operate. This point is discussed further in Sections 3.3 and 3.4.

At low sensation levels (around 10–20 dB SL) the loudness of a complex sound is roughly independent of bandwidth. This also is easy to explain. At these low levels firing rates change relatively rapidly with intensity, and so does loudness. The loudness of a single critical band changes almost in direct proportion to intensity, so that increasing the spread of energy from one to two critical bands,

Introduction to the Psychology of Hearing

for example, produces two component bands each half as loud as the original sound (Scharf, 1970). The total loudness will thus equal that of the original single band, so that loudness is independent of bandwidth. At very low sensation levels (below 10 dB), if we distribute the energy of a complex sound over a wide range of frequencies, then at no frequency will the individual components be audible, nor will there be enough systematic effect on the nervous system for the widely separate components to interact to make the whole audible. Accordingly, near threshold, loudness must decrease as the bandwidth of a complex sound is increased from a sub-critical value. As a consequence, if the intensity of a complex sound is increased slowly from a sub-threshold value, the rate of growth of loudness will be greater for a wide-band sound than for a sub-critical sound.

3.2.2 *The threshold of complex sounds*

When two tones with a small frequency separation are presented together, a sound may be heard even when either tone by itself is below threshold. Gässler (1954) measured the threshold of multitone complexes consisting of evenly spaced sinusoids. As the number of tones in a complex was increased, keeping the total energy constant, the threshold remained constant, until the overall spacing of the tones reached the critical bandwidth. Thereafter the threshold increased. Similar results are found when bands of noise are substituted for the multitone complexes. These results indicate that the energies of the individual components in a complex sound will summate, in the detection of that sound, provided that the components lie within a critical band. However, components lying outside the critical band contribute little to the detectability of the sound. The concept of the critical band as the frequency range over which the ear will integrate energy has been used in the theory of signal detection (see Section 3.7) to describe data on both masked and absolute thresholds.

3.2.3 *Two-tone masking*

Zwicker (1954) measured the threshold of a narrow band of noise, of centre frequency f, in the presence of two tones, with frequencies on either side of f. Increasing the frequency difference, Δf, between the two tones had no effect on the threshold of the noise until Δf

reached a critcal value, when the threshold fell sharply. The values of Δf at which the transition occurred correspond closely with the critical band estimates obtained in other experiments.

3.2.4 *Sensitivity to phase*

The sounds which we encounter in everyday life often change in frequency and amplitude from moment to moment. In the laboratory the perception of such sounds is often studied using either frequency-modulated or amplitude-modulated sine waves. Such waves consist of a carrier frequency (a sine wave) upon which some other signal is impressed. In amplitude modulation (AM) the carrier's amplitude is varied so as to follow the magnitude of a modulating sine wave, while the carrier frequency remains unchanged. In frequency modulation (FM) the carrier's instantaneous frequency is varied in proportion to the modulating signal's magnitude, but the amplitude remains constant. The two types of waveform are illustrated in Figure 3.4.

Although these waveforms are quite complex, they are periodic, and so they can be analysed into a series of sinusoidal components. For an AM wave the results of the analysis are very simple: the spectrum contains just three frequency components. If the carrier frequency is f_c and the modulating frequency is g, then the three components are $f_c - g, f_c$ and $f_c + g$ (all in Hz). For an FM wave the spectrum is somewhat more complex, but if the depth of modulation (which is related to the size of the frequency swing) is small, thcn the FM wave can also be considered as consisting of three components: $f_c - g, f_c$ and $f_c + g$. Under some conditions an AM wave and an FM wave may have identical frequency components, the only difference between them being in the relative phase of the components. If, then, the two types of wave are perceived differently, the difference is likely to arise from a sensitivity to the relative phase of the components.

Zwicker (1952) measured one aspect of the perception of such stimuli, namely the just detectable amounts of amplitude or frequency modulation, for various rates of modulation. He found that for high rates of modulation, where the frequency components are widely spaced, the detectability of FM and AM was equal when the components in each type of wave were of equal amplitude. However, when all three components fell within a critical band, AM was more

99

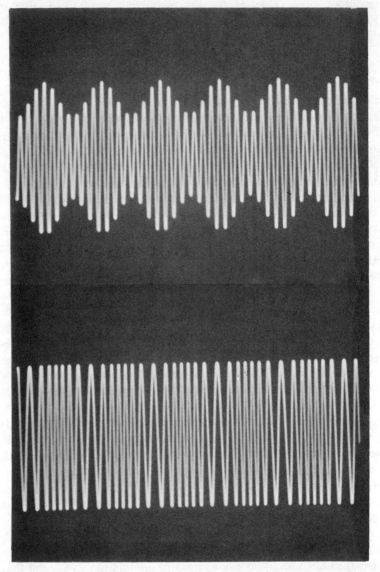

Figure 3.4 Waveforms of an amplitude-modulated wave (upper) and a frequency-modulated wave (lower).

easily detectable than FM. Thus it appears that we are only sensitive to the relative phase of the components, in the detection of modulation, when those components lie within a critical band.

It is not at present clear whether this finding can be generalised to the perception of supra-threshold levels of modulation, or to other aspects of our sensitivity to phase. Indeed there is some evidence to the contrary. For example, it has been shown that subjects can respond to cues associated with phase changes between octave complexes (e.g. 500 Hz and 1000 Hz), in which the components are separated by more than a critical band (Lamore, 1972; Raiford and Schubert, 1971). Further work is needed to clarify the nature of these discrepancies, and to determine the applicability of the critical band concept to the phase sensitivity of the ear.

3.2.5 *The discrimination of partials in complex tones*

According to Ohm's (1843) acoustical law, the ear is able to separate out the individual sinusoidal components in a complex periodic sound. This ability is called 'frequency analysis', although that term is also used to describe a more general and basic process entering any psychoacoustic task involving frequency resolution. Plomp (1964) used a complex tone with twelve sinusoidal components to investigate the frequency-analysing power of the auditory system. The listener was presented with two comparison tones, one of which was of the same frequency as a partial in the complex; the other lay halfway between that frequency and the frequency of the adjacent higher or lower partial. The listener had to judge which of these two tones was a component of the complex. Plomp used two types of complex: a harmonic complex containing harmonics 1 to 12, where the frequencies of the components were integral multiples of that of the fundamental, and a non-harmonic complex, where the frequencies of the components were mistuned from simple frequency ratios. He found that for both kinds of complex only the first five to eight components were discriminable. If it is assumed that a partial will only be distinguished when it is separated from its neighbour by at least one critical band, then the results can be used to estimate the critical band. Above 1000 Hz the estimates obtained in this way coincide with other critical band measures. Below 1000 Hz the estimates are about two-thirds as large. When Plomp repeated the experiment using a two-tone complex, he found that the partials could be distinguished at smaller frequency separations than were found for multitone complexes.

Thus, while the results are roughly in line with other measures of critical bandwidth, there are discrepancies, especially at low frequencies. It is possible that the analysis of partials from a complex sound depends in part on factors other than pure frequency resolution. Some indication of this is given by the work of Soderquist (1970). He compared musicians and non-musicians in a task very similar to that of Plomp, and found that the musicians were markedly superior. This result could mean that musicians have narrower critical bands, but this is unlikely if the critical band reflects a basic physiological process, as is generally assumed (Scharf, 1970). It seems more plausible that some other mechanism is involved in this task and that musicians, because of their greater experience, are able to make more efficient use of this mechanism. Haggard (1974) also reports comparisons of different measures of the critical bandwidth, and suggests that discrepancies at low frequencies may be explained by the intervention of non-critical band mechanisms. This problem is discussed more fully in the following section.

3.3 THE NATURE OF THE CRITICAL BAND AND MECHANISMS OF MASKING

Figure 3.5 shows the critical bandwidth as a function of centre frequency. It may be seen that data from a large number of experiments produce remarkably similar estimates of the critical bandwidth. It seems that sound energy within a critical band is treated differently from energy outside the band, and that sub-critical stimuli are treated similarly with respect to masking, loudness and threshold. The mechanism is analogous in some ways to a system of band-pass filters; stimuli within the same filter are not treated separately, whereas stimuli falling in different filters are. There do appear, however, to be discrepancies from this general rule, particularly, as was mentioned above, in the case of sensitivity to phase and the analysis of partials from a complex sound.

The locus of the critical band mechanism is still uncertain, although the frequency-resolving power of the basilar membrane is almost certainly its initial basis. One problem is that the patterns of vibration observed on the basilar membrane are quite broad in comparison with the normal critical band estimates (von Békésy, 1960).

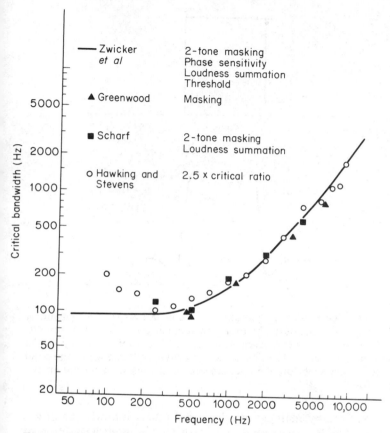

Figure 3.5 The critical bandwidth as a function of frequency. The results of four entirely separate sets of measurements are shown. Notice the similarity of the different estimates. From Scharf (1970), by permission of the author and Academic Press, London.

von Békésy suggested that lateral inhibition (presumably in the neural network in the cochlear partition) caused the broad patterns of excitation to be transformed into sharply circumscribed areas of sensation surrounded by areas of inhibition. He called the combined area of sensation and inhibition the neural inhibitory unit, and Zwislocki (1965) calculated the size of this unit to correspond to the critical band. Carterette, Friedman and Lovell (1969) attempted to provide psychoacoustic evidence for such lateral inhibition in an experiment using bands of noise with very sharp spectral edges.

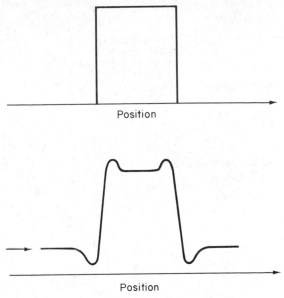

Figure 3.6 Schematic representation of the neural response to a band of light. The upper part of the figure is the luminance profile of the stimulus and the lower part is the neural response, which is influenced by lateral inhibition. Notice the elevation of neural activity at the edge of the band and the reduction below the spontaneous level (indicated by the arrow) just outside it.

They reasoned by analogy with the visual situation in which a bright band of light is viewed against a dark background. The edges of such a band look brighter than the centre of the band, while the area of the background adjacent to the band looks darker than the rest of the background. This phenomenon is generally ascribed to lateral inhibition; receptors responding to the edge of the band will be inhibited less than receptors responding to the centre of the band, owing to the adjacent dark area, thus producing a 'bright' band. The 'dark' band in the background can be explained similarly by assuming a spread of inhibition from receptors responding to the edge of the light band. The situation is illustrated schematically in Figure 3.6. The 'bright' and 'dark' bands are known as Mach bands.

Carterette and co-workers argued that neural responses to the noise bands should be enhanced in those neurones responding to the edges of the noise band, by analogy with the 'bright' bands in

104

the visual situation. They suggested that this enhanced neural response to the noise should be revealed by an elevated masked threshold for tones whose frequencies coincided with the edges of the band, and they claimed to find exactly this effect. However, similar work by Rainbolt and Small (1972) failed to show any edge effects, and the consensus of opinion is that such experiments do not provide clear evidence for lateral inhibition. Nevertheless, effects of the type predicted by Carterette and co-workers do occur with masking which is not simultaneous (see Section 3.4).

If the critical band mechanism does depend on some neural inhibitory process, then it is reasonable to expect that the process would take several milliseconds to become effective; work on lateral inhibition in other sensory systems has indicated a time constant of about 30 ms. Some critical band experiments have indicated that the time required for the critical band to be effective is considerably less than this. For example, Port (1963) found that measures of loudness summation for short-duration stimuli (as short as 1 ms) give the same value for the critical band as is found at long durations. Other experimental results, involving thresholds (e.g. Zwicker, 1965a, b; Srinivasan, 1971) have been taken to indicate a wider critical band at short durations. At the present time the reasons for the discrepancies are not entirely clear. Zwicker and Fastl (1972) in a review of this area concluded that the results which have been taken to indicate a wider critical band at short durations can, in fact, be explained in other ways, so that it is not necessary to assume a development of the critical band with time. Rather, the critical band mechanism may be viewed as a system of filters which are permanently and instantaneously present. If this is the case, then it seems unlikely that any neural inhibitory process operates in the formation of the critical band, unless that process operates at a very early stage in the processing of the acoustic stimulus and involves very few neural synapses.

It is clear that Fletcher's original conception of the critical band as a system of filters, each responding to a limited range of frequencies, has not been modified in any fundamental way by more recent work. However, Fletcher's ideas about the mechanisms involved in masking have not stood up so well. He suggested that masking involved the saturation of certain channels (i.e. critical bands) by the masking stimulus. Once a channel was saturated, the response of that channel would not change when a signal was presented, so that the signal would be masked. Thus for Fletcher masking involved a 'pre-emption' of certain channels by the masking stimulus. This concept of masking does not fit in very well with the known properties of the auditory nervous system. For example, even a tone at a very low level (say 20 dB SL) can have a masking effect on tones of adjacent frequencies, while at the same time it is unlikely that such a tone would produce any neural saturation.

Other workers have modified Fletcher's ideas, but still base their explanations of masking on the amounts of activity evoked by the stimuli at various points along the basilar membrane (these or their later neural transformations are often called excitation patterns; see Chapter 1). Consider, for example, the case of a tone presented together with a wide-band white noise. The noise will produce a pattern of excitation along the basilar membrane without any well-defined peaks, and the tone will produce a pattern of excitation with a maximum at some point. It has been suggested that the tone will be detected when the amount of excitation at some location exceeds by a fixed amount the excitation at surrounding locations, i.e. when there is a detectable maximum in the overall pattern of excitation (see, for example, Schubert, 1969; Greenwood, 1961). This theory also has certain difficulties associated with it. When a tone is at its masked threshold, the level of the tone is about 4 dB *less* than the level of the noise in the critical band around the tone. This is the average discrepancy between critical ratios and critical bands; 4 dB corresponds to a power ratio of about 2.5:1. The combined excitation of tone signal and noise masker will produce an overall level in that critical band which is about 1.5 dB above the level in surrounding critical bands. While this figure is comparable with the intensity difference limen (DL) for pure tones (i.e. for sounds within the same critical band), it is not clear whether such accuracy could be achieved for the comparison of levels in different critical bands. An important point to remember here is that results may depend on the type of task used. In a two-alternative forced-choice (2AFC) task the observer is presented with two successive bursts of noise, and is asked to say which burst contained the tone. Under these conditions the subject would be able to compare the levels in the *same* critical band on two successive occasions. Thus performance might differ markedly from that in a task where the subject is presented with a single burst of signal plus noise or noise alone and is asked to say whether a tone is present or not.

Attempts have also been made to explain the masking of one pure tone by another in terms of the interaction of excitation patterns at some peripheral level. von Békésy (1963) pointed out that there could conceivably be two different modes of interaction. One would involve the *summation* of the excitation patterns of the masker and the masked tone (in a way similar to that described for a tone plus noise); whether masking occurred or not would be determined by the magnitude of the local secondary maximum in the excitation patterns. The second mode would involve a *subtraction* of the patterns of excitation, the excitation produced by the masked tone being decreased by the presence of the masker. However, as von Békésy (1963) pointed out, this second mode of interaction could only occur if the auditory system had some way of distinguishing between the nerve impulses evoked by signal and those evoked by the masker. When the masker and the target tone have different frequencies, variations in their relative intensities would produce changes in the position of the maximum in the joint excitation pattern, and, hence, on a place theory (discussed more fully in Chapter 4) would change the subjective pitch. Both of the modes of interaction discussed by von Békésy would predict such pitch shifts, but the shifts predicted would be in opposite directions. Summation of the excitation patterns would produce a pitch shift towards the masker, while subtraction would produce a shift away from the masker. Psychophysical experiments, using both tones and bands of noise as masking stimuli (Webster and Muerdter, 1965; Terhardt and Fastl, 1971), have failed to give a clear decision in favour of either mode, and in every case the pitch shifts observed have been much smaller than predicted by von Békésy (1963) on the basis of a place mechanism. We should note, however, that two tones do not generally produce a stationary pattern of excitation on the basilar membrane. Changes in the excitation pattern as a function of time may well have an effect on masked thresholds and on pitch (see, for example, Zwicker and Schutte, 1973).

An alternative way of considering masking is provided by the 'capture effect' which was described briefly in Chapter 1 (Section 1.4). To recapitulate: In response to a single pure tone neural firings tend to occur at a particular phase of the stimulating waveform, so that intervals between nerve firings are multiples of the period of that tone. This phase-locking occurs for stimulating frequencies up to about 5 kHz. In response to two tones which are non-harmonically related, discharges may be phase-locked to one tone, or the other, or both tones simultaneously. Which of these occurs is determined by the intensities of the two tones and their frequencies in relation to the response area of the fibre. When phase-locking occurs to only one tone of a pair, each of which is effective when presented alone, the temporal structure of the response may be indistinguishable from that which occurs when that tone is presented alone. Further, the discharge rate may be similar to the value produced by that tone alone. In other words, the dominant tone appears to 'capture' the response of the neurone.

It is possible that this 'capture effect' underlies the masking of one tone by another. Clearly, the results we have described apply only to the responses of single auditory nerve fibres, and their application to the responses over an ensemble of fibres is still uncertain. However, it seems reasonable to suggest that a tone (with a frequency below 5 kHz) will be masked when its presence produces no detectable effect on the time pattern of nerve impulses evoked by the stimulus as a whole. This account of masking is, of course, only valid for tones which are presented simultaneously to the same ear, since it is only under these conditions that the 'capture effect' operates. Other factors must be involved in non-simultaneous masking and dichotic or central masking.

An explanation of masking in terms of temporal patterns of neural firing could account for the discrepancies observed by Plomp (1964) in human subjects' abilities to analyse partials from two-tone complexes and multitone complexes. As was mentioned earlier, Plomp found that a partial could only be 'heard out' from a multitone complex if that partial were separated from neighbouring partials by about one critical band. However, for a two-tone complex the partials could be identified for separations less than this. If we consider the patterns of vibration evoked by these stimuli on the basilar membrane (see Figure 3.7), we see that for a partial within a multitone complex there is no point on the basilar membrane which is responding uniquely to that partial, at least for the higher partials in the complex; the pattern of vibration at each point results from the interference of a number of components. For a partial in a two-tone complex there will be certain points on the basilar membrane whose temporal patterns of vibration *do* correspond uniquely (or almost so) to one or the other of the component tones. Thus the patterns of nerve firings derived from these regions could signal

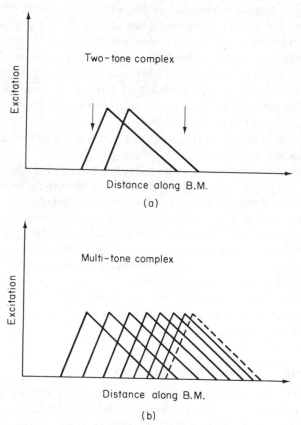

Figure 3.7 Idealised representations of the excitation patterns along the basilar membrane (B.M.) for (a) a two-tone complex and (b) a multitone complex. Notice that for the two-tone complex there are places, indicated by the arrows, responding primarily to one or the other of the component tones.

the individual pitches of the component tones. This explanation, in terms of the time pattern of the nerve impulses evoked by the stimuli at various points along the basilar membrane, can account for the differences which are found between two-tone complexes and multi-tone complexes, and can also explain why the critical band estimates derived from Plomp's results deviate from those found by other methods (e.g. loudness summation) for low frequencies.

The masking of a tone by wide-band noise can also be interpreted in terms of temporal processes. In this case the tone would be detected when the pattern of nerve firings derived from an area on the basilar membrane showed a certain level of temporal regularity or periodicity. A similar explanation could account for the detection of a tone at absolute threshold; here the temporal regularity would be detected against a background of spontaneous neural firings. This temporal theory interpretation is supported by the physiological evidence (Hind, 1972) that phase-locking is actually observed at intensities below that required to raise the average discharge rate above spontaneous level.

It should be emphasised that it is still a matter of debate whether the auditory system is capable of utilising the timing information which is available in the pattern of nerve firings (see, for example, Whitfield, 1970). This will be discussed more fully in Chapter 4. For the moment it is clear that neither masking nor the phenomena associated with the critical band involve simple processes, and that in seeking explanations of these we should be prepared to consider a number of possible underlying mechanisms. It may well be that different types of explanations are appropriate under different conditions, and that no single explanatory principle will account for all of the experimental data.

3.4 NON-SIMULTANEOUS MASKING

'Simultaneous masking' is the term used to describe those situations we have discussed where the masker is present throughout the relatively long signal. Time effects in masking have also been studied fairly intensively. Short signals, often called 'probes', are presented at various times in relation to the masker. Three basic types of masking can be distinguished: (1) backward masking, in which the probe precedes the masker (also known as pre-stimulatory masking); (2) per-stimulatory masking, in which a relatively short probe is presented at various times during the on-time of the masker, and the course of masking as a function of time is determined; and (3) forward masking, in which the probe follows the masker (also known as post-stimulatory masking). Forward masking is just one of three conceptually distinct processes which may affect the threshold of a probe presented after another sound; the other two are adaptation and fatigue, which were discussed in Chapter 2. Forward masking is distinguished from adaptation and fatigue primarily by the range of time intervals involved, although the separation is rarely clear-cut. Forward masking is generally considered to be limited to a time of a few hundred milliseconds after the cessation of the masker.

We summarise below the main features of non-simultaneous masking, based on the work of Elliot (1971) and others.

(1) The nearer in time to the masker that the signal occurs, the more is its threshold elevated. This always occurs when the masker level is above 40 dB SL. Sometimes the curve relating threshold to the time delay between masker and signal is U-shaped, showing 'sensitisation', or a lowering of threshold, when the signal occurs soon after a 'not too intense' stimulus of similar frequency characteristics (Moore and Welsh, 1970).

(2) More backward than forward masking occurs for very short time intervals between the signal and the masker (we will denote such a silent interval by the symbol Δt). Also, in simultaneous masking the threshold is more elevated for a signal occurring soon after the onset of the masker than for a signal occurring later.

(3) Most backward or forward masking occurs within about ± 100 ms of the masker onset or termination.

(4) Masking is more pronounced when signal and masker are presented to the same ear, although dichotic listening also produces backward masking and small amounts of forward masking.

(5) The amount of masking increases with increasing masker duration for Δt between 1 and 20 ms, but is approximately independent of masker duration outside this range.

(6) Both backward and forward masking are influenced by the relation between the frequencies of the signal and the masker (just as in the case of simultaneous masking). Frequency selective backward masking may occur over time intervals up to 100 ms. In forward masking the threshold may be elevated for frequencies outside a narrow masker band, when the masker is of short duration (25 ms). This is another example of threshold experiments indicating a wider critical band at short durations (see Section 3.3).

(7) Increments in masker intensity do not produce corresponding increments in amount of forward and backward masking. For example, if the masker level is increased by 10 dB, the masked threshold may only increase by 3 dB. This contrasts with simultaneous masking, where, at least for wide-band maskers, threshold usually corresponds to a constant signal-to-masker ratio.

(8) The masking of a probe signal in a short temporal gap between two maskers is greater than would be predicted from a simple summing of the amounts of backward and forward masking, i.e. the two types of masking interact.

The basis of forward and backward masking is still not clear. Forward masking could be explained in terms of a reduction in sensitivity of recently stimulated cells, or in terms of a persistence in the pattern of neural activity evoked by the masker, although other factors are probably involved. Backward masking is more difficult to explain, since it is the interference of a later masker with a signal which is physically completed, although clearly the processing of that signal cannot be complete. Further, backward masking occurs over time intervals which are longer than those required for the development and decay of the travelling wave pattern along the basilar membrane. Thus physiological processing of the stimulus is also implicated; the excitation pattern from one signal, or the central activity involved in its processing, must persist for some time after the cessation of that signal if the later activity produced by a more intense signal can overtake and obscure that from the earlier signal.

Elliot (1967) has suggested that a number of distinct but interacting phenomena are required to explain the data summarised in points (1)–(8). One such phenomenon is the time-dependent organisation of *frequency contours*, for stimuli containing narrow band(s) of frequencies. According to Elliot, frequency contours are representations, at one or more levels in the auditory system, of the edges of a band or bands. This idea is closely related to von Békésy's (1960) concept of the inhibitory unit, which was discussed earlier. The contours would correspond to the boundaries between areas of excitation and areas of inhibition. Elliot suggested that a time-dependent organisation of the frequency contours would explain the finding that in forward masking by brief narrow-band maskers threshold may be elevated for frequencies outside the narrow masker band; the narrow-band masker would initially produce a wide-band representation within the auditory system, and the narrow-band characteristics would only develop after a certain processing time had elapsed. It is not clear whether this explanation is appropriate. The reader may recall that attempts to demonstrate lateral inhibition effects in simultaneous masking have proved inconclusive (Carterette *et al.*, 1969; Rainbolt and Small, 1972). This problem is analogous in many ways to that of the time course of the development of the critical band, and some experiments indicate that the critical band is present even for stimuli of short duration (see above).

Another class of phenomena discussed by Elliot is that of on- and off-effects. These could be either neural or mechanical in origin. Duifhuis (1973) has suggested that at short Δt values (less than about 20 ms) the dominant component in both forward and backward masking results from a temporal overlap of cochlear responses. That is to say, the vibrations evoked by the first stimulus on the basilar membrane will not have completely died away before the second stimulus arrives. If this is the case, then backward and forward masking effects at short Δt values should be more pronounced for low frequencies than for high (de Boer, 1969a, b). A comparison of the results of different workers (Elliot, 1962; Gruber and Boerger, 1971; Patterson, 1971) reveals that this is indeed the case. Further, Duifhuis (1971) has demonstrated that for short Δts the masked threshold is affected by the relative phase of the masker and the signal, as would be expected if there were a temporal overlap of the patterns of vibration on the basilar membrane (although the phase effect could occur at higher levels in the auditory system if phase is preserved).

While at least part of the observed masking at short Δts might be explained in terms of peripheral mechanisms, such as fatigue and temporal overlap of vibration patterns, it is clear that higher neural levels must be invoked to account for the results at long Δts. This is suggested not only by the length of time over which the effects last, but also by the fact that backward and forward masking effects are observed in dichotic listening. Further, these effects occur both for simple stimuli, such as tones and bands of noise (Deatherage and Evans, 1969), and for complex stimuli, such as speech sounds (Darwin, 1971). Darwin's results show that the extraction of complex auditory features from a target can be disrupted by the subsequent dichotic presentation of a sound sharing certain features with the target.

The data summarised in points (1)–(8) indicate that there is a lack of symmetry between forward and backward masking effects. For example, more backward than forward masking occurs at very short Δts, for both monaural and dichotic presentations of the masker and the probe. This lack of symmetry, and the fact that effects greater than would be predicted from a simple summation are observed in situations involving both forward and backward masking, indicate that different underlying processes may be involved in these two types of masking. Again, effects exceeding simple summation have been found both for tone stimuli (Elliot, 1969; Patterson, 1971) and for speech stimuli (Dirks and Bower, 1970).

In summary, the empirical phenomena of forward and backward masking are now fairly well known, although the exact masking functions obtained depend to some extent on the specific experimental situation used. The nature of the underlying processes is less well understood. Contributions from a number of different sources may be important, these contributions being related to different neural levels in the auditory system. At the peripheral level temporal overlap of patterns of vibration may be important at short Δt values. Also at this level some sort of temporary fatigue effect may play a role in forward masking. At higher neural levels a persistence of the excitation pattern evoked by the stimulus seems to be required. The nature of the interactions between the excitation patterns of the signal and masker remains uncertain.

3.5 EVIDENCE FOR LATERAL INHIBITION FROM NON-SIMULTANEOUS MASKING

We described earlier Rainbolt and Small's (1972) replication of the work of Carterette *et al.* (1969), measuring the thresholds of sinusoids in bands of noise with sharp spectral edges. Rainbolt and Small concluded that there were no edge effects indicative of any form of lateral inhibition. Houtgast (1972) has argued that simultaneous masking is not an appropriate tool for detecting the effects of lateral inhibition. Its use is based upon the assumption that when the nervous activity corresponding to some frequency region is influenced by lateral inhibition (e.g. at the edges of a band-pass noise with a sharp cut-off in frequency), the masked threshold for a test tone would also be affected near that frequency. Houtgast argued that, in simultaneous masking, the masking stimulus and the test tone are processed simultaneously in the same channel. Thus any inhibition in that channel will affect the nervous activity caused by both the test tone and the masking noise. In other words, the signal-to-noise ratio in a given frequency region will be unaffected by lateral inhibition, and thus the threshold of the test tone will remain unaltered.

Houtgast suggested that this difficulty could be overcome by presenting the masker and the test tone successively (i.e. by using a forward masking technique). If lateral inhibition does occur, then

its effects will be seen in the forward masking threshold curve provided that: (1) in the chain of levels of neural processing the level at
which the lateral inhibition occurs is not later than the level at which
most of the forward masking effect arises; (2) the inhibition built
up by the masker has decayed by the time that the test tone is
presented (otherwise the problems described for simultaneous masking will be encountered).

Houtgast used a repeated-gap masking technique, in which the
masker was presented with a continuous rhythm of 150 ms on, 50 ms
off. Probe tones, with a duration of 20 ms, were presented in the gaps.
He used as maskers high- and low-pass noises with sharp spectral
cut-offs (96 dB/octave), and also a sound with a spectral peak (tone
plus noise). The masking curves obtained showed edge effects,
similar to Mach bands in vision; both 'bright' band and 'dark'
band effects could be discerned. No such effects were observed in the
case of simultaneous masking. Thus forward masking does reveal
the type of effects which an inhibitory process would produce.

Houtgast also noted a very remarkable feature of the repeated-
gap technique; when the bursts of probe tone are just above threshold,
they sound like a continuous tone. Only at higher levels of the probe
tone is the perception in accord with the physical time pattern,
namely a series of tone bursts. Houtgast called the level of the probe
tone, at which its character changed from pulsating to continuous,
the pulsation threshold. He showed that the existence of such a
pulsation threshold is a very general feature of alternating stimuli, and
is not restricted to the alternation of two stimuli with a frequency
component in common. However, the phenomenon does not occur
when the masker contains no frequency component in the neighbourhood of the probe tone. He suggested the following interpretation of
the phenomenon: 'When a tone and a stimulus S are alternated
(alternation cycle about 4 Hz), the tone is perceived as being continuous when the transition from S to tone causes no (perceptible)
increase of nervous activity in any frequency region.' In terms of
patterns of excitation this suggests that 'the peak of the nervous
activity pattern of the tone at pulsation threshold level just reaches
the nervous activity pattern of S'. Given this hypothesis, the pulsation
threshold for a test tone as a function of frequency can be considered
to map out the apparent spectrum of the stimulus S (i.e. its excitation
pattern) on the nervous activity level. The pulsation threshold curve
will thus reflect both the frequency-analysing properties of the

mechanical part of the inner ear and the effects of lateral inhibition.

We may conclude that Houtgast's results do show clearly the types of effects which would be expected if inhibitory mechanisms were operating. The neural level at which the effects occur remains uncertain. Houtgast points out that simultaneous masking patterns and envelopes of the patterns of vibration in the basilar membrane (Johnstone *et al.*, 1970) have similar slopes on the low-frequency side (about 100 dB/octave), whereas the slopes obtained by the pulsation threshold or repeated-gap masking techniques resemble those found for the tuning curves of primary auditory neurones (200–500 dB/octave). Thus it is possible that the direct masking curve represents the stimulus at a pre-inhibitory stage, possibly on the basilar membrane level, whereas the pulsation threshold curve represents the stimulus at a nervous activity level, a post-inhibitory stage. The similarity between the pulsation threshold curves and the tuning curves of primary auditory neurones would presumably indicate that the inhibition occurs at an early stage in the processing of the signal.

It is still not clear that inhibitory processes are responsible for the effects described by Houtgast. Indeed there are a number of difficulties facing this theory. Firstly, it may be inappropriate to attempt to account for forward masking purely in terms of peripheral activity patterns, since processing at levels higher than the auditory nerve is almost certainly involved. Secondly, results from the pulsation threshold technique seem to be strongly influenced by the exact timing of the stimuli, so that quantitative evaluation of the slopes of masking curves is difficult. Thirdly, the processes underlying the observed neural effects are still uncertain, so that most workers now prefer to use the term 'suppression' rather than 'inhibition', to avoid unnecessary implications about a particular class of physiological mechanisms (Sachs, 1971: pp. 149–151).

Whether or not lateral inhibition occurs, the fact remains that individual neurones are more sharply tuned than would be predicted from the 'tuning' curves on the basilar membrane. Recent data on the patterns of vibration on the basilar membrane (e.g. Rhode, 1971) have indicated a sharper tuning than was found by von Békésy (1960), but some discrepancy remains between the neural and the mechanical data. Thus either the travelling wave envelope does not represent the ultimate input to the neural system (as has been suggested by a number of workers; see, for example, Tonndorf, 1970) or there is some further mechanism which provides a sharpening of responses. The possibility of a 'second filter' after the basilar membrane is at present the subject of intensive research. Robertson and Manley (1974) reported that the normal sharp tuning observed in auditory neurones can be altered by reducing the oxygen supply to the animal. Slowing the rate of ventilation made the tuning curves less sharp and at the same time decreased sensitivity. These changes were reversible. Similar effects have been reported by Evans (1975), who also investigated the effects of ototoxic agents such as cyanide and frusemide. It appears that the normal sharp tuning of auditory nerve fibres depends upon a mechanism which is physiologically vulnerable, and that the loss of the sharp tuning is accompanied by an elevation in threshold. Evans and Harrison (1975), using the drug kanamycin to produce selective damage of the outer hair cells, concluded that the threshold and tuning properties of auditory nerve fibres are dependent on the integrity of the outer hair cells even though the great majority of fibres innervate only inner hair cells.

Evans (1975) has pointed out that in fibres affected by anoxia or ototoxic drugs the tuning properties approximate those of the basilar membrane. Thus, in the absence of the physiologically vulnerable 'second filter', the tuning properties in the auditory nerve can be accounted for in terms of basilar membrane mechanics. Evans has suggested that damage of a similar nature may occur in human deafness of cochlear origin, and that loss of the 'second filter' can account for the widening of the critical band, the loudness recruitment and the degradation of speech perception which occurs in such cases.

Robertson (1976) has reported that conditions which lead to a loss of sharp tuning in primary auditory neurones also result in the disappearance of two-tone suppression. Thus the non-linearity associated with the suppression appears to be connected with the sharpening process. It is possible that this non-linearity is also involved in the generation of combination tones of the type $2f_1 - f_2$ (Duifhuis, 1976). These combination tones are discussed in Section 4.3.

3.6 GENERAL CONCLUSIONS

A great many of the phenomena discussed in this chapter can be understood in terms of the frequency-resolving power of the auditory system, at least part of which results from the mechanical action of the basilar membrane. The different frequency components in a complex stimulus are separated out to a certain extent, so that only components within a certain frequency range interact in any way. The general properties of this frequency analysis are summarised in the critical band concept; listeners' responses to complex stimuli will differ depending on whether the components of the stimuli fall within one critical band or are spread over a number of critical bands. The critical band is revealed in experiments on masking, loudness summation and threshold. Other types of experiment reveal discrepancies from this general rule. Thus a sufficiently intense tone may mask another for frequency separations *greater* than the critical band. On the other hand, the separate partials in a two-tone complex can be correctly identified for frequency separations *less* than the critical band.

The processes underlying the masking phenomenon are still not well understood. Two general types of explanation have been suggested. One involves the detection of differences in the *amounts* of activity at various points in the auditory system. The other involves the detection of changes in the *time pattern* of neural activity at various points in the auditory system. The relative importance of these two types of mechanism remains to be determined, but some dependence on the particular task employed is almost certain to be found. The temporal mechanism would only operate in tasks involving the detection of periodic or quasi-periodic stimuli. It is possible that temporal mechanisms may be responsible for the differences in the critical band function obtained by methods involving pure frequency-place analysis (e.g. loudness summation) and methods which might involve temporal analysis (e.g. tone–tone masking, noise–tone masking). The former show a curve which flattens out between 2 kHz and 500 Hz, while the latter show a curve which continues to decrease down to about 200 Hz.

The processes underlying the phenomena of forward and backward masking are also poorly understood. A number of stages can be distinguished in these processes; these stages must be related to different levels of neural activity, but what these levels are, and the nature of the interactions between the excitation patterns of the signal and the masker, remain to be determined. Houtgast's experiments, involving repeated-gap masking and the pulsation threshold were interpreted by him as indicating the action of inhibitory processes, analogous to the suppression effects which have been observed in primary auditory neurones. However, the mechanisms underlying these suppression effects are not known, and it seems premature to draw too close a connection between the psycho-physical and the neurophysiological data; non-simultaneous masking almost certainly depends in part on neural activity at levels higher in the auditory system than the auditory nerve.

The frequency selectivity shown in primary auditory neurones may depend in part on the action of a filtering mechanism operating after the basilar membrane. This 'second filter' appears to be physiologically vulnerable, and its properties are currently the subject of intensive research.

We see, then, that the critical band may be conceived as a filter whose characteristics reflect the frequency-analysing properties of the basilar membrane and also possibly some further sharpening process. This sharpening process seems to be established at an early stage in the auditory system.

3.7 APPENDIX: SIGNAL DETECTION THEORY

3.7.1 *Introduction*

A great deal of Chapters 2 and 3 has been concerned with the measurement of thresholds. Classically, a threshold has been considered as that intensity of a stimulus above which it will be detected and below which it will not. It has been known for many years that this viewpoint is unsatisfactory; if the intensity of a stimulus is slowly increased from a very low value, there is no well-defined point at which it suddenly becomes detectable. Rather there is a range of intensities over which the subject will sometimes report a signal and sometimes will not. Thus a plot of percentage correct detections against the intensity of the stimulus (such a plot is called a psychometric function) typically has the form shown in Figure 3.8. A further problem is that a subject's performance may be altered by, for example, changing the instructions, while at the same time the stimulus itself has remained unaltered. Thus it seems that factors not directly associated with the discriminability of the signal may influence the observer's performance. Signal detection theory provides a means of separating factors relating to criterion, motivation, bias, etc., from factors relating to purely sensory capabilities. It also enables us to account for the fact that responses may vary from trial to trial even when an identical stimulus is presented on each trial.

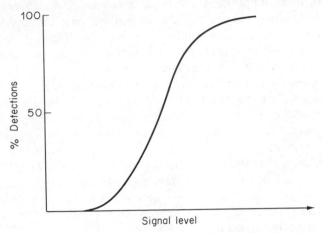

Figure 3.8 A typical psychometric function showing how the percentage of detections of a signal varies with signal level.

3.7.2 *The basic idea of signal detection theory*

The theory assumes that decisions are based upon the values of some internal variable x. The nature of x is not precisely specified. One might consider it to correspond to the 'sensory impression' evoked by the stimulus, or one might think of it in more physiological terms; x might correspond to the number of neural firings occurring in some particular channel during the presentation time of the stimulus. The important point is that such a variable exists, and that its average value is monotonically related to the intensity of the stimulus, i.e. increases in the intensity of the stimulus will, on average, increase the value of x. The second important assumption of the theory is that the value of x will fluctuate from trial to trial, even though the same signal is presented. This variability may arise from two sources. The signal may actually be presented against a variable background, such as a noise, so that fluctuations in physical intensity occur. Alternatively, or in addition, the source of the variability may be neural; most neurones exhibit a pattern of random firings in the absence of external stimulation, so that the presence of a stimulus will be signalled as an increase in firing rate superimposed upon this pattern of random activity. Even in neurones with low spontaneous activity the response to a fixed stimulus may vary from trial to trial.

120

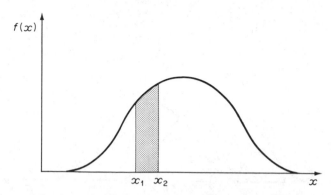

Figure 3.9 A probability density function. The probability of x lying between the two values x_1 and x_2 is given by the shaded area under the curve. The total area under the curve is 1.

We see then that although the average value of x will depend on whether a signal is present or absent, on any given trial the observer will never be asbolutely sure that a signal has occurred, because of the inherent variability of x. Of course, if we make the signal sufficiently intense, the increase in x will be large compared with this variability, and thus the uncertainty becomes vanishingly small. But for faint signals the best that the observer can do is to make a guess on the basis of the value of x which occurred on that particular trial.

To proceed further, we have to make certain assumptions about the distribution of x. Since x is a random variable, we cannot predict its exact value on any trial, but we can specify the probability that x will fall within a specified range of values. One way of doing this is to plot a probability density function, $f(x)$. The expression $f(x)$ simply implies that f is a function of x. A probability density function, $f(x)$, is defined in such a way that the probability of x lying between x and $x + dx$ (where dx represents a small change in the value of x) is equal to $f(x)$ multiplied by dx. A probability density function is illustrated in Figure 3.9. The probability that x lies between two values, x_1 and x_2, is given by the area under the curve between these two points. Since, on any given trial, some value of x must occur, the total area under the curve is equal to 1.

Consider the situation where an observer is given a series of trials, on some of which a signal is present and on some of which it is

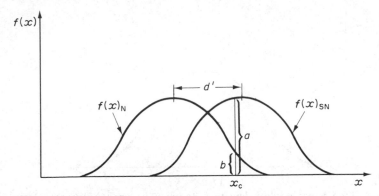

Figure 3.10   The two distributions (probability density functions) which occur in response to 'noise' alone [$f(x)_N$], and 'noise' plus signal [$f(x)_{SN}$]. The separation between the means of the two curves, denoted by d', gives a measure of the discriminability of the signal. The criterion value is labelled x_c, and the ratio of the heights of the curves at x_c, namely a/b, gives the likelihood ratio, β.

absent. To describe this situation we need to specify two probability density functions; one describes the distribution of values of x when no signal is present (this is often denoted by $f(x)_N$, the suffix N referring to the 'noise', either external or neural, which gives rise to this distribution), and the other describes the distribution of values of x where a signal does occur (often denoted $f(x)_{SN}$). It is usually assumed that these two distributions are normal, or Gaussian, and that they have equal variances. There are some theoretical reasons for making this assumption, but normal distributions are also chosen because results are easier to handle in terms of the mathematics involved. The distributions are usually plotted with standard deviation units along the abscissa; in other words, they are scaled so as to have a standard deviation of unity. They will appear as in Figure 3.10. For each of these two distributions the mean value of x corresponds to the peak in the distribution, and the separation between the two peaks, denoted by d', gives a measure of the separation of the two distributions, and thus of the discriminability of the signal.

The theory assumes that the subject establishes a cut-off point corresponding to a particular value of x, which we may denote x_C. If, on any given trial, the value of x which actually occurs is greater than x_c, the subject will report that a signal was present; otherwise he will report no signal. Just what value of x_c is chosen will depend upon the instructions to the subject, the probability of a signal, the system of rewards of punishments, previous experience, etc. Since the exact nature of x is not specified, we cannot assign a number to x_c. To overcome this problem a new quantity is introduced—the likelihood ratio, β. This is defined as the ratio of the heights of the two distributions at x_c, i.e. as $f(x_c)_{SN}/f(x_c)_N$. In other words, the quantity β is equal to the likelihood ratio that a central effect of magnitude x_c arose from the presentation of a signal plus noise as opposed to noise alone. In Figure 3.10 β would be equal to a/b. In contrast to d' which gives us a pure measure of the discriminability of the signal, β is related to the criterion of the subject and gives us a measure of changes in motivation, etc., independent of any changes in sensory capability.

In a given experiment we can measure the proportion of times the subject responds yes when a signal was present, $P(H)$ (this is called the probability of a hit), and the proportion of times he responds yes when a signal is absent, $P(F)$ (this is called the probability of a false alarm). From these proportions, and given our assumption that the distributions are normal and of equal variance, it is easy to calculate the values of d' and β. A simple example of how this is done is given in Welford (1968: p. 33). In practice the situation is even easier than this, since tables exist giving the values of d' and β for any given values of $P(H)$ and $P(F)$.

The major advantage of signal detection theory, then, is that it enables us to separate changes in performance related to purely sensory factors from changes related to motivational or criterion factors. Notice that this can only be done by measuring the proportion of false alarms as well as the proportion of hits. Classical methods of determining thresholds, ignoring as they did the former measure, were not able to achieve this separation. We should note further that according to this theory there is no such thing as a sensory threshold; any given intensity of a signal presented to an observer will have associated with it a certain value of d', but there will be no particular value of the intensity which corresponds to threshold.

In practice, if we are interested in comparing the discriminability of different types of signals, we can measure the intensity of the signal needed to produce a particular value of d'. Alternatively, we can use a task which attempts to eliminate the effects of bias or criterion, so that threshold can be arbitrarily defined as corresponding to a particular percentage correct. One type of task which has proved useful in this respect is the two-alternative forced-choice (2AFC) task, in which there are two observation intervals, only one of which contains the signal. The theory assumes that for each observation interval a particular value of x occurs, and that the subject simply chooses the interval in which the largest value of x occurs. It turns out to be the case that results in a 2AFC task can be simply related to those in a 'single interval' task; 76 per cent correct in 2AFC corresponds to a d' of 1.

3.7.3 *Application of signal detection theory to theories of masking*

Although we do not need to specify the nature of x in order to apply this theory, many workers have considered what x might be. The question is equivalent to enquiring about the nature of the processes involved in masking—what features of a signal, or of its representation at a neural level, enable us to distinguish it from a masking stimulus. Some workers have considered that the masking of a tone by a noise can be explained purely in terms of the statistics of the stimuli; in other words, the variability of x arises primarily from the inherent variability of the stimuli rather than from any 'internal variability'. An example of this type of approach is given by the work of Jeffress (1964). He assumed that all stimuli are filtered, so that only a narrow band of frequencies in the noise contribute to the masking of the tone, i.e. he assumed a critical band mechanism. After this is an envelope detector, and following this a criterion device. Jeffress showed that this model gave a good fit to much of the data obtained in detection experiments. Other workers (e.g. Swets *et al.*, 1962) have assumed that stimulus energy rather than the stimulus envelope is the feature on which decisions are based. Again, however, it is necessary to assume a critical band mechanism.

This class of models, in which variability in the signals rather than variability in the observer limits performance, may be considered as describing different types of 'ideal observer'. These models have never been intended as complete descriptions of the human observer, since it is clear that interval variability does play a significant role; human observers rarely if ever achieve the performance levels which would be predicted as 'ideal'. This does not mean, however, that they are of no value. Rather, they provide 'a class of normative models with which the observer's performance can be compared' (Tanner and Sorkin, 1972).

4

Pitch Perception and Auditory Pattern Perception

4.1 INTRODUCTION

We will now consider some perceptual aspects of the complex sounds introduced in Chapter 1. In that chapter pitch was defined as that attribute of auditory sensation in terms of which sounds may be ordered on a musical scale, i.e. that attribute in which variations constitute melody. Pitch is related to the repetition rate of the waveform of a sound; for a pure tone this corresponds to the frequency, and for a harmonic complex tone to the fundamental frequency. There are, however, exceptions to this simple rule, as we shall see later. Since pitch is a subjective quality, it cannot be measured directly. Assigning a pitch value to a sound is generally understood to mean specifying the frequency of a pure tone having the same subjective pitch as the sound.

Timbre is a sensation or class of sensations related more generally to the quality of a sound. It was defined by the American Standards Associations (1960) as 'that attribute of auditory sensation in terms of which a listener can judge that two sounds similarly presented and having the same loudness and pitch are dissimilar'. Thus differences in timbre will enable us to distinguish between the same note played on, say, the piano, the violin and the flute. Schouten (1968) has suggested that five major physical parameters influence timbre: (1) spectral envelope—the distribution of energy as a function of frequency; (2) tonal versus noise-like character; (3) time variations in the waveform envelope; (4) change in any of the previous parameters; (5) the nature of the preceding sounds. Plomp (1970) has suggested a more restricted definition of timbre as 'that attribute of sensation in terms of which a listener can judge that two steady complex tones having the same loudness, pitch and duration are dissimilar'. This reduces timbre to dependence upon the spectra of the stimuli (i.e. their harmonic content) and on the relative phases of the components, the former being the more important factor. For example, complex tones with strong lower harmonics (up to the 6th) sound mellow, whereas sounds with strong harmonics beyond the 6th or 7th sound sharp and penetrating.

In a situation involving the recognition of musical instruments listeners may use any or all of the factors listed by Schouten. The initial transients seem to be particularly important. We may view Plomp's definition as one of convenience, to include only properties that are at present relatively well understood.

The primary aim of this chapter is to discuss the mechanisms underlying the perception of pitch and timbre. As we shall see, a good deal more work has been done on pitch than on timbre. Later on in the chapter we shall discuss the problem of how we are able to 'hear out' individual instruments in the orchestra and how we recognise the types of auditory patterns which occur in music and speech.

4.2 THEORIES OF PITCH PERCEPTION

The classical place theory of hearing has two distinct postulates. The first is that the stimulus undergoes some sort of spectral analysis in the inner ear, so that different frequencies (or frequency components in a complex stimulus) excite different places along the basilar membrane. The second is that the pitch of a stimulus is related to the pattern of excitation produced by that stimulus; for a pure tone the pitch is generally assumed to correspond to the position of maximum excitation. The first of these two postulates is now almost universally accepted, and has been confirmed in a number of independent ways, including direct observation of the movement of the basilar membrane (see Chapter 1). The second is still a matter of dispute. An alternative to the place theory, which will be called a temporal theory, suggests that the pitch of a stimulus is related to the time pattern of the neural impulses evoked by that stimulus. Nerve firings tend to occur at a particular phase of the stimulating waveform, and thus the intervals between successive neural impulses will approximate integral multiples of the period of the stimulating waveform. The reader will recall that in Chapter 3 the possible role of this temporal information in masking was discussed.

Neither of these theories can account for our perception of pitch over the whole of the audible range; von Békésy (1960) has shown that the patterns of vibration on the basilar membrane do not shift as a function of frequency for frequencies below 50 Hz. On the other hand, the synchrony of nerve impulses to stimulus cycles has not been observed for frequencies above 5 kHz (Rose *et al.*, 1968). Thus there is a large range of frequencies over which either or both of these mechanisms could be operating. A difficulty for the place theory arises when we consider complex tones. These produce patterns of excitation along the basilar membrane which do not show a single well-defined maximum; rather there is a distribution of excitation, whose maximum, or maxima, may not correspond to the fundamental component. However, the perceived pitch, in general, still corresponds to this component. We shall discuss later how the place theory may be modified to account for this.

4.2.1 *The perception of pure tones*

In this section we shall discuss theories which attempt to explain how we perceive and discriminate pure tones. However, the ultimate aim is to produce a theory which is consistent with the data for both pure and complex tones. We shall see later on that there are close relationships between these two types of data, and that these relationships point to a unified framework in which to order the data. The main topics which we shall discuss in relation to pure tones are the size of the frequency difference limen (the smallest detectable change in frequency, abbreviated DL), and changes in the size of the DL and other aspects of our perception of pure tones which occur as a function of frequency. We shall see that these changes can provide important insights into the ways in which complex tones are perceived.

A basic problem for any theory of hearing is to account for the remarkably small size of the frequency DL; for a frequency of 1 kHz and at a moderate intensity a change of about 3 Hz can be detected, and with practice some observers achieve even smaller DLs. This is a particular problem for the place theory, since the patterns of vibration which have been observed on the basilar membrane seem much too broad to account for this acuity.

Several different types of hypotheses have been advanced to account for the sharpening which appears to be necessary. von

127

Békésy (1960) has suggested that the discrimination may be achieved through a process similar to that involved in Mach bands in vision; a process of lateral inhibition results in an accentuation of contours. We discussed in Chapter 3 the possibility that such sharpening plays a role in the formation of the critical band. Huggins and Licklider (1951) suggested various ways in which sharpening could be achieved by mechanical processes, and several other mechanical solutions have been advanced since. They all involve rather detailed mathematical arguments about the exact form of the pattern of vibrations on the basilar membrane and the way in which these are transformed into neural impulses. For example, Tonndorf (1970) has suggested that a shearing motion on the basilar membrane is the ultimate mode of mechanical input to the hair cells and that sharpening occurs in the shear wave transformation.

It is well worth considering theories which attribute part of the sharpening to mechanical processes, because the tuning curves in primary auditory neurones are sharper than the corresponding tuning curves for the patterns of vibration on the basilar membrane (see Section 3.5). However, contrary to what is often supposed (and written), there is little evidence for progressive sharpening at higher points in the auditory system (Møller, 1972). Furthermore, the tuning curves of individual neurones still seem to be too broad to account for the size of the frequency DL.

Zwicker (1970) has attempted to account for the DL size in terms of changes in the 'excitation pattern' evoked by the stimulus. The shapes of the 'excitation patterns' are inferred from data on the masking of tones by narrow bands of noise (see Chapter 3), and the patterns at different centre frequencies have similar shapes if they are plotted with critical bands along the abscissa rather than frequency. According to Zwicker's model, a change in frequency will be detected whenever the excitation on the steeply sloping low-frequency side of the excitation pattern changes by 1 dB or more (see Figure 4.1). Maiwald (1967) has shown that the steepness of this slope is almost independent of the level and of the frequency of the exciting tone, and has a value of 27 dB/Bark (a Bark is a unit of one critical band). Thus Zwicker's model would predict that the frequency DL at any given frequency should be a constant fraction (1/27) of the critical bandwidth at that frequency.

The frequency DLs obtained by the modulation method (e.g. Shower and Biddulph, 1931) do conform fairly well to these predic-

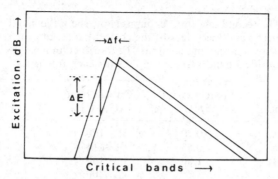

Figure 4.1 Schematic representation of the patterns of excitation evoked by two tones of slightly different frequency. According to Zwicker, the patterns will have a similar shape, regardless of frequency, when they are plotted in terms of critical bands rather than frequency. The greatest difference in excitation for the two patterns occurs on the steeply sloping low-frequency side. A change in excitation, ΔE, of 1 dB or more is assumed to be detectable.

tions. This method involves shifting the frequency of the test tone up and down about four times per second and determining the minimum detectable frequency shift. However, Henning (1966) has shown that the method is unreliable, especially at high frequencies, since here frequency changes may be accompanied by correlated loudness fluctuations; the response of headphones on real ears is generally very irregular at high frequencies, and there is also a loss of absolute sensitivity of the observer at high frequencies (see the right-hand half of Figure 2.1). These loudness fluctuations may provide observers with usable cues in the detection of frequency modulation. A generally better method is the two-interval forced-choice (2IFC) task, in which a subject is presented on each trial with a pair of successive tone pulses and is asked to judge whether the first or the second had the higher pitch. This is varied randomly from trial to trial, and the frequency DL is usually taken as that frequency separation between the pulses for which the subject achieves 75 per cent correct.

Some results using this method are given in Table 4.1 (data from Moore, 1974). The table also shows the critical band values given by Scharf (1970) and the ratio of the critical band to the frequency difference limen, which according to Zwicker's model should be approximately constant. It may be seen that the ratio varies by a

Table 4.1. The second and third columns show the frequency DLs (mean of three subjects) and the values of the critical bandwidth for each of the frequencies shown in the first column. The fourth column shows the value of the ratio (critical band)/(frequency DL) for each frequency

Frequency	Frequency DL, Δf (Hz)	Critical band (CB) (Hz)	CB/Δf
250 Hz	0.70	100	143
500 Hz	0.83	114	137
1 kHz	1.80	160	89
2 kHz	3.8	300	79
4 kHz	12.9	660	51
6 kHz	38	1130	30
8 kHz	96	1650	17

factor of over 8 to 1 in the range considered. Further, at low frequencies the subjects are doing considerably better than would be predicted on the basis of this model.

Further evidence on this question has been presented by Moore 1972, 1973a). He measured the frequency DL for tone pulses of various durations. For a short-duration tone pulse the frequency spectrum contains energy at frequencies other than the nominal frequency, f, of the tone pulse. This effect is quite a general one; whenever a stimulus is altered from its steady state (e.g. by switching on or off), energy is spread or 'splattered' into adjacent frequency regions (see Section 1.2). The shorter the tone pulse is made, the wider the range of frequencies over which the energy is spread (see Figure 4.2). Below some critical duration the slope of the spectral envelope will be less than the slope of the excitation pattern evoked by a long-duration pure tone. Thus, if Zwicker's model is correct, this physical slope will limit performance at short durations. Given these assumptions, and assuming that a 1 dB change is detectable, it may be shown that

$$\Delta f \times d > 0.24$$

where Δf is the frequency DL for a tone pulse of duration d. (See Moore, 1973a, for details of the calculations involved.) The results showed that at short durations observers did better than predicted for all frequencies up to 5 kHz. At about this frequency the DLs showed a sharp increase in value (see Figure 4.3). This is in accord with previous findings (Henning, 1966). Further, when the results

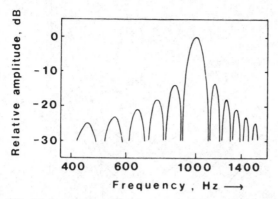

Figure 4.2 The spectrum of a short tone pulse of frequency 1 kHz, with a rectangular envelope and a duration of 10 ms. With shortening duration the energy spreads over a wider range of frequencies, and the slope of the envelope of the spectrum becomes less steep.

are plotted in terms of the relative increase in DL for each frequency (Figure 4.4), a clear kink is observed between 4 and 6 kHz.

These results are consistent with a change in mechanism at about 5 kHz. It seems that a model based on shifts in excitation patterns is inadequate to explain the results for frequencies below this. The inadequacy of this type of model has been confirmed by other experimental results (Feth, 1972; Moore, 1972, 1973a–c). Other types of place model have been suggested (e.g. Corliss, 1967; Siebert, 1968, 1970; Henning, 1967), but none of these is completely satisfactory in explaining either the DL size at short durations or the changes which occur at about 5 kHz. It seems that we must seek some alternative mechanism, the obvious candidate being the temporal theory. The loss of neural synchrony at about 5 kHz would explain the changes which occur at this frequency, and would also explain certain other changes in the way that pure tones are perceived. One such change is a loss of 'musical pitch' for pure tones above 5 kHz; a sequence of such tones does not produce a sense of melody. This has been confirmed experimentally by experiments involving octave matches (these become erratic when the higher tone lies above 5 kHz) and by experiments involving musical transposition. For example, Attneave and Olson (1971) asked subjects to reproduce sequences of tones (e.g. the NBC chimes) at different points along the frequency scale. Their results showed an abrupt breaking

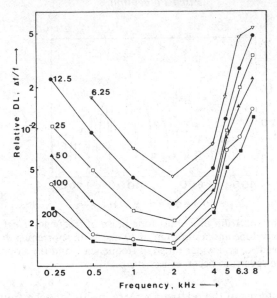

Figure 4.3 Relative frequency DLs, $\Delta f/f$, as a function of frequency. The parameter is duration of the tone pulses in msec. Both scales are logarithmic. Notice the sharp increase in the size of the DLs which occurs around 5 kHz.

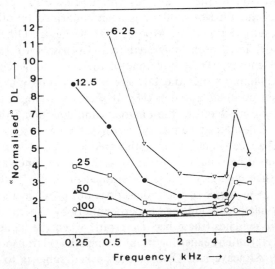

Figure 4.4 This figure shows the same data as Figure 4.3, plotted in terms of 'normalised' DLs. For each frequency the 'normalised' DL is obtained by dividing the DL for a given duration by the DL for duration 200 ms. Plotting the results in this way enables us to see more clearly the effect of shortening duration. Notice the 'kink' in the curves at about 5 kHz.

point at about 5 kHz, above which transposition behaviour was erratic.

It seems quite clear that some sort of change occurs at around 5 kHz, and the fact that this change occurs at the same frequency at which the phase-locking of neural impulses ceases to exist is highly suggestive. However, there are still considerable difficulties involved with a temporal model. One of these is that so far there has been no evidence of a physiological mechanism which could carry out the time measurements involved with sufficient accuracy. The DL size at 1 kHz requires that a time interval of 1 ms be measured with an accuracy of about 3 μs. When we consider that there is a certain 'jitter' in the initiation of nerve impulses, which, according to de Boer (1969a), has a standard deviation of about 100 μs for a 1 kHz tone, the problem becomes even more acute; the mechanism must also be required to 'average' over time and over different auditory nerve fibres. However, the absence of physiological or anatomical evidence for an appropriate time-measuring mechanism should not necessarily be discouraging, since similar problems exist in explaining our ability to resolve interaural time differences of a few microseconds, in localisation and lateralisation judgements (see Chapter 5), yet clearly we do have this ability (Tobias, 1972).

von Békésy (1963) suggested a further problem associated with a temporal theory, that 'an increase in firing rate should produce not only an increase in loudness, but, if pitch is assumed to be connected with firing rate, a rise in pitch as well'. Thus it should be difficult for the auditory system to separate out pitch and loudness. This problem disappears if we assume that pitch is not connected with firing rate *per se* but with the time intervals between nerve firings, or bursts of nerve firings. Consider, for example, a neurone which is firing, on average, on every fourth cycle of the stimulus. If the intensity of the stimulus is now increased, the firing rate may increase, so that the neurone fires on every third cycle, but the firings remain locked to a particular phase of the stimulating waveform, and the intervals between firings remain integral multiples of the period of that waveform. In fact nerve firings tend not to occur as regularly as this (Rose *et al.*, 1968), but the physiological evidence indicates that phase-locking is maintained over a wide range of intensities, so that the timing information in a single fibre, or over a group of fibres, will convey the same pitch regardless of changes in the overall rate of firing.

The two mechanisms we have been discussing are not, of course, mutually exclusive; it is likely that place information is available over almost all of the auditory range but that temporal mechanisms allow greater efficiency in certain types of task for frequencies up to 5 kHz. If this interpretation is correct, we see that a true sense of musical itch is only obtained for frequencies where a temporal mechanism is operating, and it is interesting to note that the highest orchestral notes have frequencies lying just below 5 kHz.

4.2.2 *The pitch of complex tones*

As was stated earlier in this chapter, the classical place theory has difficulty in accounting for the way in which we perceive complex tones. For such tones the pitch does not, in general, correspond to the position of maximum excitation on the basilar membrane. A striking example of this is provided by the 'phenomenon of the missing fundamental'. Consider, as an example, a sound consisting of short impulses (clicks) occurring 200 times per second. This sound has a low pitch, which is very close to the pitch of a 200 Hz pure tone, and a sharp timbre. It may be shown to contain harmonics with frequencies 200, 400, 600, 800 . . ., etc., Hz. However, it is possible to remove (electronically) the 200 Hz component, and it is found that the pitch does not alter; the only result is a slight change in the timbre of the note. Indeed, we can eliminate all except a small group of high harmonics, say 1800, 2000 and 2200 Hz, and the low pitch still remains, although the timbre will now be markedly different.

Schouten (1940) called this low pitch associated with a group of high harmonics the residue. He pointed out that the residue is distinguishable, subjectively, from a fundamental component which is physically presented or from a fundamental which may be introduced (at high sound pressure levels) by non-linear distortion in the ear. Thus it seems that the perception of a residue pitch does not require activity at the point on the basilar membrane which would respond maximally to a pure tone of similar pitch. This is confirmed by a demonstration of Licklider (1956) which showed that the low pitch of the residue persists even when the low-frequency channels are 'saturated' with low-frequency random noise. Thus it seems that low pitches may be perceived via those neural channels that normally respond to the high- or middle-frequency components of a signal.

A number of models have been proposed to account for the residue effect and for certain other phenomena associated with the perception of complex tones (see below). These models may be divided into two broad classes. The first class (which we will call 'pattern recognition' models) assumes that the pitch of a complex tone is derived from neural signals corresponding to more primary sensations, such as the pitches of the individual partials. The second class of models involve the assumption that pitch is based on time interval measurement. In particular, it has been suggested that the pitch of a complex tone is related to the time interval between peaks in the fine-structure of the signal close to adjacent envelope maxima (Schouten, Ritsma and Cardozo, 1962). If nerve firings tend to occur at these peaks, then this time interval will be present in the time pattern of neural impulses. Let us examine each class of model in more detail.

4.2.3 *Pattern recognition models*

Thurlow (1963) suggested that pitch arises on the basis of place information (i.e. according to the spatial pattern of activity on the basilar membrane), but the response is mediated by vocal activity. This vocal activity may be overt or subliminal, or involve only auditory imagery. Thurlow's mediation hypothesis suggests that the subject produces either overtly or covertly a comparison signal whose fundamental frequency is adjusted so that its harmonics coincide with those of the complex tone presented. The perceived pitch will correspond to that fundamental frequency. A similar type of theory, but one not requiring an active matching process, has been suggested by Whitfield (1967, 1970). He suggests that a complex tone gives rise to a series of active groups of nerve fibres in the central auditory pathway, separated by groups of inactive fibres. Although each of these groups corresponds to one of the partials of the complex, we do not normally hear these as such. Rather, we hear a unitary experience of a complex sound to which we ascribe a pitch. The total pattern in the auditory pathway corresponds to this pitch. Clearly, there is a whole group of patterns to which the same pitch is attributed by the system. Whitfield suggests that these patterns are learned as a result of our exposure to harmonic complex sounds (which in nature usually include the fundamental) from the moment the auditory system commences to function. The absence or distortion of a part of the pattern (e.g. by removing the fundamental) will not entirely destroy the normal sensation. The mechanism will try for the best fit among known patterns; the interpretation put on the available data is that which is 'most likely'.

Both of these theories are inadequate in the sense that they do not state exactly what components of a complex stimulus are important in determining the pitch of a complex as a whole. For example, Whitfield (1970) says that 'pitch is related to some weighted average of all the components', and that 'the way in which this average is taken is complex'. To see why this point is important let us consider the experiments of Schouten *et al.* (1962). They investigated the pitch of amplitude-modulated sine waves, which may be shown to contain just three sinusoidal components. Thus a 2000 Hz sine wave (the 'carrier' frequency) modulated 200 times per second contains components at 1800, 2000 and 2200 Hz, and has a pitch which is similar to that of a 200 Hz sine wave. This would be predicted by either of the theories discussed above. Consider now the effect of shifting the 'carrier' frequency to, say, 2040 Hz. The complex now contains components at 1840, 2040 and 2240 Hz. This stimulus would be very unlikely to occur naturally; how will the subject choose the appropriate matching pattern? One possibility is that he makes his judgement on the basis of the spacing between adjacent partials, in which case the pitch would be altered. On the other hand, the partials correspond to the 46th, 51st and 56th harmonics of a 40 Hz fundamental, and so an appropriate matching stimulus would have the same pitch as a 40 Hz sinusoid. In fact, the perceived pitch, in this particular case, corresponds roughly to that of a 204 Hz sinusoid. In addition, there is an ambiguity of pitch, so that matches around 185 Hz and 227 Hz are also found.

While it is possible to explain these results in terms of *post hoc* arguments about the weighting of the various components, it seems that Whitfield's model is not sufficiently precise to allow us to predict the pitch of any given complex tone. A model which does not suffer from this defect has been proposed by Walliser (1968, 1969a–c). His model does not specify the mechanisms by which the pitch of a complex tone will be perceived, but provides a rule for determining the 'periodicity pitch', or residue pitch, of complex tones. There are two parts to the rule: (1) The pitch corresponding to the frequency difference between neighbouring partials (i.e. the envelope repetition rate) is approximately determined. This may be inferred from the pitch differences between adjacent partials (for high repetition rates where partials are well separated), or it may be determined from 'the roughness sensation' (for low repetition rates where the partials are closely spaced). The 'roughness sensation' seems to be related to fluctuations in the envelope of the stimulus. (2) A subjective sub-harmonic of the lowest present partial is found, such that the pitch of this sub-harmonic lies as close as possible to the pitch determined in (1).

To illustrate the working of the rule consider again the example discussed above, of a complex tone with components at 1840, 2040 and 2240 Hz. The envelope repetition rate, which is the same as the spacing between adjacent partials, is 200 Hz. The lowest partial is 1840 Hz, and the sub-harmonic of this which lies closest to 200 Hz is 204.4 Hz (1840 divided by 9). This corresponds closely to the perceived pitch.

Terhardt (1972a, b) has modified and elaborated this model, suggesting that a residue pitch will always be a sub-harmonic of a dominant partial rather than simply the lowest partial. By dominant he means 'partials which are resolvable', i.e. which can be heard out from the complex as a whole. Terhardt suggests that these dominant partials lie in the frequency region between 500 and 1500 Hz. According to this model, then, a residue pitch will only be heard when at least one partial can be analysed from the complex. When the partials are too close together in frequency, they will no longer be resolvable, and no residue pitch will be heard.

Terhardt (1974) has recently extended this model to include a learning phase. Repeated stimulation with harmonic complex tones (speech sounds) enables the mechanism to 'learn' the spectral cues corresponding to such tones. After the learning phase is completed, stimulation by a single pure tone will produce pitch cues corresponding to several sub-harmonics of that tone. When a harmonic complex tone is presented, the pitch cues corresponding to these sub-harmonics will coincide at certain values, with the largest number of coincidences occurring at the fundamental. Thus the overall pitch will correspond to that of the fundamental. This version of the model requires that more than one harmonic can be analysed from the complex.

An alternative model, although one still dependent on the resolution of individual frequency components in a complex tone, has been presented by Goldstein (1973). In this model the pitch of a complex tone is derived by a central processor which receives information only on the frequency, and not on the amplitude or phase, of individual components. The processor presumes that all stimuli are periodic and that the spectra comprise successive harmonics (which is the usual situation for naturally occurring sounds). The processor finds the harmonic series which provides the 'best fit' to the series of components actually presented. For example, if we present components at 1840, 2040 and 2240 Hz (as in the experiment by Schouten and co-workers described above), then a harmonic complex tone with a fundamental of 204 Hz would provide a good 'match'; this would have components at 1836, 2040 and 2244 Hz. The perceived pitch is in fact close to that of a 204 Hz sinusoid. According to this model, errors in estimating the fundamental occur mainly through errors in estimating the appropriate harmonic number. In the above example the presented components were assumed by the processor to be the 9th, 10th and 11th harmonics of a 204 Hz fundamental. However, a reasonable fit could also be found by assuming the components to be the 8th, 9th and 10th harmonics of a 226.7 Hz fundamental, or the 10th, 11th and 12th harmonics of a 185.5 Hz fundamental. Thus the model predicts the multimodal pitch matches which are actually observed for this stimulus. The extent to which such multimodal pitch matches occur will depend upon the accuracy with which the frequencies in the stimulus are represented at the input to the central processor.

All of the models which we have described in this section depend on the spectral resolution of individual components in the stimulus. It is predicted that no 'residue' pitch will be heard if no frequency components can be analysed or 'heard out' from the complex. We will discuss the experimental evidence relating to this in a later section. The mechanism by which individual partials would be analysed from a complex tone has not generally been specified, although Terhardt (1972a, b) has suggested that this could operate via an extended place principle, and that the basic determinant of the pitch of a complex sound is the spatial pattern of activity on the basilar membrane. This is not a necessary assumption for these models. Indeed Goldstein (1973) was careful to state that '... the concept that the optimum processor operates on signals representing the constituent frequencies of complex-tone stimuli does not necessarily imply the use of tonotopic or place information *per se* as the measure of frequency. For example, temporal periods of pure tones are not ruled out as the measure of frequency.' As we saw in the section on pure tones, there is quite good evidence that temporal mechanisms play a part in our perception of pure tones, at least for frequencies up to 5 kHz. Thus it is likely that the analysis of partials from a complex tone, and the determination of their pitches, relies at least in part on temporal mechanisms. Given this assumption, these models could still hold, but the basic data on which they operated would be the temporal patterns of firing in different groups of auditory neurones.

We shall discuss later some of the experimental evidence which is relevant to these models. Let us now turn to the second main type of model—the 'temporal' model.

4.2.4 *Temporal models*

Consider again the examples of a pulse train of repetition rate 200/s, containing harmonics at 200, 400, 600, ... Hz. The lower harmonics in this sound will be analysed into effectively separate locations on the basilar membrane, and the timing of the neural firings derived from these locations will relate to the frequencies of those harmonics rather than to the repetition rate of the complex as a whole. However, the patterns of vibration on the basilar membrane corresponding to the higher harmonics will overlap to some extent, so that the waveform on the basilar membrane will result from the interference of a number of harmonics, and will show a periodicity the same as that of the input waveform. The timing of neural impulses derived from such a region would then relate to the repetition rate of the original input waveform. This is illustrated in Figure 4.5 (see also Figure 1.9).

These considerations lead to a theory whose development is mainly due to Schouten (1940, 1970). We summarise below the major points of his theory.

(1) The ear analyses a complex sound into a number of components each of which is separately perceptible.

(2) Some of these components correspond with individual partials present in the input waveform. These components have a pure tone quality.

(3) One or more components may be perceived which do not correspond with any individual sinusoidal oscillation, but which are a collective manifestation of some of those oscillations which are not or are scarcely individually perceptible. These components (residues) have an impure, sharp tone quality.

139

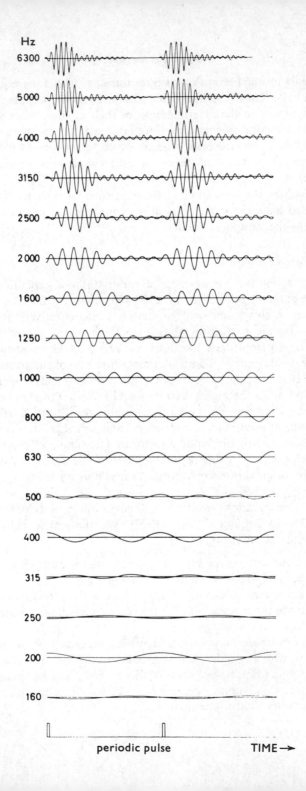

(4) The ear ascribes a pitch to a residue by virtue of the periodicity of the total waveform of the harmonics which are responsible for this residue.

(5) The pitch ascribed to a complex sound is the pitch of that component to which the attention, by virtue either of its loudness or of its contrast with former sounds, is most strongly drawn.

In general, the residue is the most prominent component in a complex sound, and thus the pitch of the whole sound will be given by the pitch of the residue. We see, then, how a low pitch may be signalled through those neural channels which normally respond to a high- or middle-frequency components of a complex sound.

Notice a major difference between this model and the pattern recognition models, such as Walliser's model. The pattern recognition models require that at least one partial in the complex sound should be analysable from the complex in order for a low-residue pitch to be heard, whereas Schouten's model requires that at least two harmonics are interacting in order for the residue to be heard. And according to Schouten's model, a residue pitch may still be heard when none of the individual components is separately perceptible.

Let us consider how Schouten's model deals with the complex tone which we discussed earlier in relation to the pattern recognition models; this contained components of 1840, 2040 and 2240 Hz. If we compare the waveform of this signal with the waveform of a signal containing components at 1800, 2000 and 2200 Hz, we see that, while the envelope repetition rates are the same, the time interval between corresponding peaks in the fine structure of the waveform is slightly different (see Figure 4.6). Since these signals contain only a narrow range of frequency components, the waveforms on the basilar membrane will not be greatly different from those of the physically presented signals; the basilar membrane will not separate the individual components to any great extent. Thus, if nerve firings tend to occur at peaks in the fine structure of the

---

Figure 4.5 A simulation of the responses on the basilar membrane to periodic impuses of rate 200 pulses per second. Each number on the left represents the frequency which would maximally excite a given point on the basilar membrane. The waveform which would be observed at that point, as a function of time, is plotted opposite that number. This figure can be compared with Figure 1.9, which represents the envelopes of responses to the same stimulus. From Plomp (1968), by permission of the author.

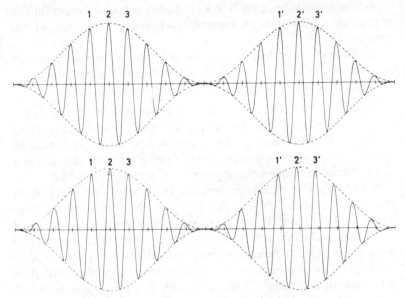

Figure 4.6 Waveforms for two amplitude-modulated sine waves. In the upper waveform the carrier frequency (2000 Hz) is an exact multiple of the modulation frequency (200 Hz). Thus the time intervals between corresponding peaks in the fine-structure, 1–1', 2–2', 3–3', will be 5 ms, the period of the modulation frequency. In the lower waveform the carrier frequency is shifted slightly upwards. Thus ten complete cycles of the carrier occur in slightly less than 5 ms, and the time intervals between corresponding points on the waveform, 1–1', 2–2', 3–3', will be slightly shorter than 5 ms. The lower waveform has a slightly higher pitch than that of the upper. From Plomp (1968), by permission of the author.

waveform close to envelope maxima, the timing of the nerve impulses will convey slightly different pitches for the two stimuli. These differences in the time pattern of neural impulses have been confirmed by Javel (1974). Notice that for the signal containing components at 1840, 2040 and 2240 Hz the time intervals between nerve firings will fall into two groups, one slightly longer than 5 ms (the period of a 200 Hz tone) and one slightly shorter than 5 ms. The shorter of these two time intervals would correspond to a pitch of about 204 Hz, which is what is normally reported, but Schouten *et al.* (1962) did also report an ambiguity of pitch, so that sometimes the perceived pitch corresponded to the longer of these two time intervals.

We see that it is necessary to refine Schouten's original theory, particularly with respect to point (4). The pitch of the residue will be determined by the time interval between peaks in the fine structure of the waveform (on the basilar membrane) close to adjacent envelope maxima. If more than one possible time interval is present, the pitch will correspond, in general, to the shortest, although sometimes ambiguity of pitch may occur. If we consider the representation of the signal on a neural level, in terms of the time pattern of nerve firings, then, just as was the case for pure tones, the time intervals between nerve firings rather than the overall rate of firing will be important. If the system were simply counting, say, the number of impulses per second, then the pitch shifts observed by Schouten and co-workers would not have occurred.

4.3 EXPERIMENTAL EVIDENCE RELEVANT TO PATTERN RECOGNITION AND TEMPORAL MODELS

Both the 'pattern recognition' models and Schouten's model give a fair description of what Schouten *et al.* (1962) called the 'first effect of pitch shift'; for an amplitude-modulated sine wave there is a slight upward shift in pitch when the carrier frequency is increased from a value which is an exact multiple of the modulation rate. This pitch shift would be predicted from the shifts which occur in the time interval between peaks in the fine-structure of the waveform close to adjacent envelope maxima (as in Figure 4.6). However, the experimental data reveal that the pitch shifts actually observed are consistently slightly larger than predicted, particularly for high harmonic numbers (when the carrier frequency is high relative to the modulation rate). The extra pitch shift, over and above the predicted 'first effect of pitch shift', was called the 'second effect of pitch shift' by Schouten and co-workers.

This 'second effect' is explained in various ways by the different models. Recall that Walliser s model required the determination of a subjective sub-harmonic of a dominant partial. Ward (1954) showed that subjective octave intervals between pure tones correspond to frequency ratios slightly greater than 2. Walliser (1968) confirmed these results and derived a scale of subjective harmonics as a function of objective harmonics. From this scale one predicts that a pitch determined as a subjective sub-harmonic will be slightly different from that calculated as an objective (i.e. mathematically perfect) sub-harmonic, and thus the 'second effect' is explained. The same reasoning can explain the finding that a periodic sound of repetition rate g periods/s is sometimes reported to have a pitch slightly different from that of a pure tone of frequency g Hz (Walliser, 1968; Terhardt, 1971). Terhardt (1972a, b) has suggested a way in which the 'octave enlargement' phenomenon could arise. He says 'our sense of musical intervals, and thereby of the octave interval, is acquired; we acquire the knowledge of harmonic relations in earliest life, when we learn to recognize and to understand speech sounds' (Terhardt, 1972c). He presents evidence showing that for a complex tone containing a fundamental and a number of harmonics, the pitch of the fundamental component is shifted slightly downwards, whereas the pitches of the 2nd and higher harmonics are shifted upwards. Thus the pitch intervals between the 1st and 2nd harmonics will be enlarged compared with the corresponding intervals for successive pure tones. By exposure to these sounds we 'learn' an octave interval which is slightly enlarged. Lindqvist and Sundberg (1971) consider this explanation unlikely, since the perceptual size of the octave, if picked out from harmonic sounds, would vary substantially, especially in vowel sounds, owing to the frequent variations of the relative levels of the two lowest partials.

An alternative explanation of the 'second effect of pitch shift' is suggested by the work of Smoorenburg (1970). He investigated the pitch perception of stimuli containing only two frequency components. Sometimes these are perceived as having a single pitch corresponding to about the (absent) fundamental, although the pitch is generally rather weak (see later for further data on this type of stimulus). Smoorenburg found that a shift of the frequencies away from a harmonic situation resulted in a pitch shift. For high harmonic numbers the shift was larger than could be accounted for either by a temporal mechanism or by a pattern recognition model, such as Walliser's. The large pitch shift, which is analogous to the second effect of pitch shift observed by Schouten and co-workers, can be explained by taking into account certain types of combination tones—in particular, those with pitches corresponding to frequencies $f_1 - K(f_2 - f_1)$, where f_1 and f_2 are the frequencies of the tones which are physically presented and K is an integer. A combination tone may be defined as a perceived tone not present in the sensations produced by the constituent components of the stimulus when they are presented singly. Combination tones of this type, and particularly those with a pitch corresponding to frequency $2f_1 - f_2$, have been shown to be audible even at moderate intensities (Plomp, 1965; Goldstein, 1967). Smoorenburg suggested that these combination tones, rather than the physically presented partials, are dominant in determining the pitch of the complex in cases where a large pitch shift occurs. He showed that when the combination tones are masked by bands of noise, the large pitch shift is diminished, although at the same time the clarity of the pitch sensation is diminished.

Notice that this type of combination tone corresponds to a lower partial of the complex which is physically presented. For example, if two tones with frequencies 1800 Hz and 2000 Hz are presented, the combination tone will have a frequency of 1600 Hz ([2 × 1800] − 2000). In the case of tones which are harmonically related, the combination tone will have a frequency corresponding to a lower harmonic of the same fundamental frequency. For primary tones of, say, 1840 Hz and 2040 Hz, the combination tone will have a frequency of 1640 Hz.

Combination tones can explain the second effect of pitch shift in terms of both Schouten's and the 'pattern recognition' models. For the former we must assume that the waveform on the basilar membrane results from the interference of physically presented partials and combination tones. For the latter we must assume that the pitch of a complex tone is determined from information relating to individual partials, combination tones included.

4.3.1 The existence region of the tonal residue

Ritsma (1962) investigated the audibility of residue pitches, for amplitude-modulated sinusoids containing three components, as a function of the modulation rate and the harmonic number (carrier frequency divided by modulation rate). Later (Ritsma, 1963) he extended the results to complexes with a greater number of components. He found that the tonal character of the residue pitch existed only within a limited frequency region. When the harmonic number was too high (above about 20), only a kind of high buzz of undefinable pitch was heard. He found, further, that some harmonics below 5 kHz had to be present for a residue pitch to be heard, and that the modulation rate had to be below about 800 Hz. Other workers (Plomp, 1967; Moore, 1973c) have found, using complex tones with a greater number of components, that residue pitches can be perceived for repetition rates up to about 1400 Hz.

Let us consider the implications of these results for the models we have been discussing. According to the pattern recognition models, a residue pitch will only be heard when at least one partial is analysable from the complex. In Chapter 3 we discussed Plomp's (1964) experiments which showed that for a partial within a multitone complex only the first 5–8 harmonics are separately perceptible, although the limit was somewhat higher for two-tone complexes. Since Ritsma (1962) found a tonal residue for complexes which only contained harmonics around the 20th, it would seem that under some conditions we can hear a residue pitch when none of the individual components is separately perceptible. We can describe these results in terms of the critical band concept; roughly speaking, components separated by a critical band or more will not interact, and will be separately perceptible, whereas components within a critical band will interact and will not produce separate pitches. Thus Ritsma's results would indicate that a low-residue pitch can be heard when the components do not fall in separate critical bands and so should not be separately perceptible. On the other hand, Terhardt (1970) investigated another aspect of the critical band phenomenon—the frequency difference between two simultaneously presented pure tones which is necessary to give a perception of two separate pitches; he found that the curve of 'pitch separation' was almost identical with the lower boundary of the 'existence region of the tonal residue'.

There are a number of difficulties in attributing a single underlying process to patterns of results, particularly graphs of performance as a function of frequency. Firstly, individual differences can be very great (see, e.g., Moore, 1973c). Thus comparing the results of different individuals in different experiments is a dubious procedure, especially when few subjects have been used. Secondly, in this particular comparison, it is not clear whether the results for two-tone complexes, or those for multitone complexes, are the more appropriate ones for comparison. Finally, it is likely that Ritsma's results were influenced by the intervention of combination tones, as has since been pointed out by Ritsma himself (1970).

Moore (1973c) carried out a series of experiments in an attempt to resolve these difficulties. He first determined that the lowest partial in a multitone complex was more easily audible than any of the other partials. In fact, it was about as easily audible as a partial in a two-tone complex. He then determined the audibility of the lowest partial in a multitone complex as a function of the frequency separation of the partials. A condition was included where a band of noise was present in the frequency region below the lowest partial. The functions relating audibility to separation were then compared with the frequency separation of the harmonics for which a complex tone produced a well-defined pitch, using the same set of subjects. Again a 'noise' condition was included, so that combination tones in the frequency region below the lowest presented partials could not influence the results. Moore found that for high harmonic numbers there was a range of conditions over which a residue pitch could be heard when none of the individual partials would have been separately perceptible. However, this range was rather small. Thus it seems that while pattern recognition models cannot explain the results for these high harmonic numbers, they could account for the results over the major part of the existence region of the residue. It does seem to be the case that residue pitches are considerably more clear when lower harmonics are present.

4.3.2 *The principle of dominance*

Taking a systematic approach to this general type of problem, Ritsma (1967a) carried out an experiment to determine which components in a complex sound are most important in determining its pitch. He used a method of conflicting pitch information, where the frequencies of a small group of harmonics were drawn apart from the rest, while at the same time these harmonics remained integral multiples of a common fundamental. The subject's pitch judgements were used to determine whether the pitch of the complex as a whole was affected by the shift in the group of harmonics. Ritsma found that 'for fundamental frequencies in the range 100 Hz to 400 Hz, and for sensation levels up to at least 50 dB above threshold of the entire signal, the frequency band consisting of the third, fourth and fifth harmonics tends to dominate the pitch sensation as long as its amplitude exceeds a minimum absolute level of about 10 dB above threshold'. This finding has since been confirmed in other ways (Ritsma, 1967b; Bilsen and Ritsma, 1967).

Thus Ritsma introduced the concept of dominance: '. . . if pitch information is available along a large part of the basilar membrane the ear uses only the information from a narrow band. This band is positioned at 3–5 times the pitch value. Its precise position depends somewhat on the subject' (Ritsma, 1970). This concept has a number of implications. Firstly, it explains why the second effect of pitch becomes more marked as the harmonic number is increased. For low harmonic numbers the partials contributing most to the pitch sensation are those which are physically present in the stimulus. For higher harmonic numbers the combination tones lie in the dominant region, and thus their contribution is more marked. Secondly, the concept of dominance may help us decide whether the components involved are interacting or are being separately analysed in the auditory system. It seems, however, that there is no clear-cut answer to this question. For the normal range of fundamentals that are used in these experiments (up to 1000 Hz), the 3rd, 4th and 5th harmonics do lie in a region where individual partials are well analysed, but the overlap of vibration patterns on the basilar membrane would also be sufficient to provide temporal information about the periodicity of the input waveform. Thus, in the dominant region, both spectral and temporal analyses would appear to be possible.

4.3.3 *Evidence for the role of central mechanisms in the perception of complex tones*

Houtsma and Goldstein (1972) conducted perhaps the first experiment which clearly demonstrates that a 'residue'-type pitch may be heard when there is no possibility of an interaction of components in the cochlea. They investigated the perception of stimuli which comprised just two successive harmonics. Subjects were required to recognise melodies corresponding to the (missing) fundamentals. Harmonic numbers were randomised from note to note, so that the subjects could not use cues associated with the pitches of individual harmonics in order to recover the melody. They found that performance was good for low harmonic numbers, but fell to chance level for harmonic numbers above about 10–12. They found further that subjects were able to identify melodies when the stimuli were presented dichotically (one harmonic to each ear). At high intensities monotic performance was superior to dichotic, whereas at low levels (20 dB SL) there was no difference between the two conditions. Houtsma and Goldstein suggested that the differences at high intensities resulted from the influence of combination tones, which would lower the effective harmonic number. They considered that if an allowance were made for the effect of combination tones, then there would be essentially no difference between the monotic and dichotic conditions.

These results cannot be explained in terms of Schouten's model, or indeed in terms of any model which requires an interaction of components on the basilar membrane (e.g. von Békésy, 1961). They imply that 'the pitch of these complex tones is mediated by a central processor operating on neural signals derived from those effective stimulus harmonics which are tonotopically resolved'. In other words, these experiments clearly indicate that the pitch of a complex tone can be mediated by some sort of pattern recognition process. However, it is not yet entirely clear that the findings apply to the pitches of complex tones in general. The pitch of a two-tone complex is not very clear; indeed, many observers do not hear a single low pitch, but rather perceive the component tones individually (Smoorenburg, 1970). Residue pitches are generally much more distinct when greater numbers of harmonics are present, and while Goldstein (1972) has reported similar results for complex tones with up to six components, no full report of this work has yet appeared. It does seem to be the case that two-tone complexes only produce a residue pitch for harmonic numbers below about 10, whereas the limit is somewhat higher for multitone complexes (Ritsma, 1962; Moore, 1973c). Thus some factor other than our ability to analyse individual components from complex tones affects the upper limit of the 'existence region'.

We conclude, then, that Houtsma and Goldstein's results clearly indicate that the pitch of a complex tone can be derived from neural signals corresponding to individual partials in the complex, at least for stimuli with low harmonics, or containing only a small number of harmonics. It is still not established whether the information about these partials is coded in terms of place or in terms of the temporal patterns of nerve firing. Houtsma and Goldstein (1972) concluded that 'all the constraints could conceivably be met by mechanisms based on either time or place information'. But it is noteworthy that residue pitches are only observed when harmonics (or combination tones) are present with frequencies below 5 kHz (Ritsma, 1962, 1963; Moore, 1973c). We saw earlier in this chapter that it is likely that temporal mechanisms are important in the perception of pure tones for frequencies up to about 5 kHz, but that above this only place mechanisms could operate. Thus residue pitches are only heard when harmonics are present in the frequency region where temporal information is available. It is apparent that a conclusion about the role of temporal information cannot be based upon any single critical demonstration, but must depend on inferences consistent with a broad range of phenomena.

4.3.4 *Pitches based upon purely timing information*

To avoid some of the difficulties associated with harmonic stimuli, a number of workers have investigated pitch sensations using stimuli which contain no spectral peaks, and which therefore would not produce a well-defined maximum on the basilar membrane. Such pitches presumably cannot arise on the basis of place information, and so provide evidence for the operation of temporal mechanisms.

Miller and Taylor (1948) presented random noise which was turned on and off abruptly, and periodically, at various rates, by an electronic switch. Provided that care is taken to eliminate switching transients (clicks), the interrupted noise will have a uniform spectrum. They reported that the noise had a pitch-like quality for interruption rates between 100 and 250 Hz. More recently Pollack (1969) has shown that subjects are able to adjust sinusoids to have the same pitch as the interrupted noise for interruption noise up to 2000 Hz. They adjust the frequency of the sinusoid to be roughly equal to the interruption rate of the noise. These experiments support the idea of a temporal analysis in the auditory system, but the pitch sensation for this type of stimulus is not very clear. This could be because the exact waveform of the noise in successive samples is different. Many subjects do not report a pitch sensation at all, although most can hear that something pitch-like changes when the interruption rate is changed. This phenomenon, that a pitch is heard more clearly if it is varied, seems to be quite a general one, and is often marked for residue pitches.

A number of experiments have been reported showing pitch sensations as a result of the binaural interaction of noise stimuli. Huggins and Cramer (1958) fed white noise from the same noise generator to both ears, via headphones. The noise to one ear went through an all-pass filter, which passed all audible frequency components without change of amplitude, but produced a phase change in a small frequency region. A faint pitch was heard corresponding to the frequency of the phase transition, although the stimulus presented to each ear alone was white noise, and produced no pitch sensation. The effect was limited to frequencies below about 1 kHz. A phase shift of a narrow band of the noise would tend to be handled as a difference in localisation by the auditory system (see Chapter 5), so that this band would be separated in subjective space from the rest of the noise. This spatial separation presumably produces the pitch-like character associated with that narrow band.

Fourcin (1970) used two noise sources, which we shall denote n_1 and n_2. n_1 was led via headphones to the two ears, producing a sound image lateralised in the middle of the head. n_2 was also fed to both ears, but the input to one ear was delayed by a certain time, τ, producing a second sound image lateralised to one side. Sometimes the observer simply heard two separate sound images, neither of which had a pitch. At other times, however, a faint pitch was heard, whose position was not well-defined, but which was generally centrally located. When the observed pitches were matched to pure tones (of frequency f), the matches lay along the line $1/\tau = 4f/3$.

Bilsen and Goldstein (1974) reported that a pitch may be perceived when just one noise source is used, presented binaurally, but with a delay at one ear. For delays shorter than about 2 ms a single noise image is reported, whose perceived position depends on the delay. For longer time delays the image remains at the side of the head and becomes more diffuse, and, in addition, 'a faint but distinct pitch image corresponding to $1/\tau$ appears in the middle of the head'. As for the pitches reported by Fourcin, the effect is an essentially low-frequency one; the highest pitch matches reported by Bilsen correspond to frequencies of about 500 Hz.

The exact mechanism which gives rise to these pitches remains to be elucidated. Since in all three of the experiments producing pitches by binaural interaction the stimuli presented to each ear separately conveyed no spectral information, timing information must be used in the creation of a central pattern of neural activity from which the pitch is extracted. In other words, information about the relative phases of components in the two ears must be preserved up to the point in the auditory system where binaural interaction occurs. We shall see in Chapter 5 that we are only able to use phase differences between the two ears in the localisation of sounds for frequencies up to about 1500 Hz, and it seems that pitches perceived by binaural interaction are limited to this region. The necessity for binaural interaction means that there is no particular obligation to regard 1500 Hz as a limit for temporal coding in general. A feature of all these pitches is that they are very faint, and indeed many observers do not hear them at all. They may arise from the operation of a mechanism which is not normally involved in pitch extraction, but is primarily concerned with the localisation of sound, and the extraction of signals from noise. Indeed, one of the models put forward to explain the pitches of these stimuli, and to account for the factor of 4/3 which was found in Fourcin's experiments (Bilsen and Goldstein, 1974), is based on Durlach's equalisation and cancellation model, which is a model designed to account for the detection of signals in noise under binaural listening conditions (see Chapter 5).

Some subjects are able to resolve the time delays as either pitches or localisation, possibly because of similarities in the prerequisite stimulus parameters. Nordmark (1970) has pointed out that there are many similarities in the systems involved in pitch and localisation, especially when periodic stimuli are used. The relationship of the faint pitches heard with noise stimuli to the much clearer pitches observed in situations where spectral information is available is not, at the moment, clear.

4.4 GENERAL CONCLUSIONS ON THE PERCEPTION OF COMPLEX TONES

It is now quite clear that the perception of a particular pitch does not depend on a high amplitude of vibration at a particular point on the basilar membrane. The pitch of complex tones will, in general, be mediated by harmonics higher than the fundamental, so that similar pitches may arise from quite different patterns of vibration on the basilar membrane. For stimuli containing a wide range of harmonics, the harmonics in a region around the 3rd, 4th and 5th will tend to dominate the pitch percept. These harmonics lie in the range where frequency resolution is possible; we can pick out the harmonics as separate entities, although we do not normally listen in this way. For stimuli containing only high harmonics, combination tones in the frequency region below the lowest harmonic may dominate the pitch percept. These combination tones behave like lower harmonics of the complex tone which is physically presented. Even allowing for these combination tones, we are sometimes able to hear a residue pitch when none of the individual partials in a complex tone are separately perceptible. Thus for stimuli containing only high harmonics the pitch may arise as a result of the interference of components at some region on the basilar membrane. The temporal pattern of nerve firings derived from such a region would depend closely upon the repetition rate of the input waveform.

For complex tones with only two components, residue-type pitches can be heard when the stimuli are presented dichotically (one harmonic to each ear). Thus the pitch of these signals must arise from a central analysis of the neural signals corresponding to the individual harmonics. This type of 'pattern recognition' process is consistent with a number of models presented in this chapter.

The basic neural data on which such a pattern recognition process would operate have not yet been clearly established. In principle, pattern recognition could proceed from a purely place mechanism of component frequency analysis, but it is likely that temporal mechanisms play a role in our perception of pure tones, and the analysis of partials from complex tones, for frequencies up to about 5 kHz. Further, residue pitches are only observed when harmonics (or combination tones) below 5 kHz are present. Thus it seems reasonable to assume that the pattern recogniser operates on data derived from the time-patterning of neural impulses in different nerve fibres. Consider, for example, the presentation of the 3rd, 4th and 5th harmonics of a (missing) 200 Hz fundamental, namely 600, 800 and 1000 Hz. In those neurones responding primarily to the 600 Hz component an analysis of time intervals between nerve firings would reveal intervals of 1.67, 3.33, 5.0, 6.67, . . . ms, each of which is an integral multiple of the period of that component (compare the interspike interval histograms in Figure 1.16). Similarly, the time intervals in the 800 Hz 'channels' would be 1.25, 2.5, 3.75, 5.0, . . . ms, while those in the 1000 Hz 'channels' would be 1, 2, 3, 4, 5, . . . ms. Notice that the time interval which is common to all of the channels is the one corresponding to the period of the fundamental (5 ms). Thus a mechanism comparing or correlating the results of an analysis of time patterns of neural firing in different groups of neurones could determine the pitch of the 'missing fundamental'.

If this is the case, then one of the great problems for any theory of hearing can be explained. The problem is this: when we listen to two or more complex tones together (e.g. two musical instruments or two vowel sounds), we do not confuse which harmonics belong to which instrument. Rather we hear each instrument or each speaker as a single source and are able to make spatial judgements about it and attend selectively to it. Broadbent and Ladefoged (1957), in an experiment using synthetic vowel sounds, showed that the normal percept of a single fused voice occurs if all the harmonics have the same fundamental frequency, even if they are fed to different ears. If the harmonics are split into two groups (formats), with different fundamental frequencies, then two separate sounds are heard. These results can be explained if we assume that the pitch of a complex tone results from a correlation or comparison of the time intervals between nerve firings in different auditory neurones. Only those channels which show a high correlation (i.e. which are linked to the same fundamental frequency) will be classified as 'belonging' to the same sound. It is difficult to see how such an analysis could be achieved by a mechanism operating only on the spatial pattern of neural activity.

Sometimes pitches can be perceived by binaural interaction, when the stimuli presented to either ear alone convey no sense of pitch. Timing information must be used in the generation of these pitches. They are, however, faint, and it is possible that they are not produced by the mechanism normally responsible for pitch perception, or that they present it with an unfavourable input.

4.5 THE PERCEPTION OF MUSIC

Since this topic could easily occupy a book of its own, we limit ourselves to discussing certain selected aspects related to the rest of this chapter. The specially interested reader is referred to Ward (1970), who gives a more comprehensive review.

4.5.1 *Octaves, musical intervals and musical scales*

It has been known for very many years that tones which are separated by an octave (i.e. where the frequencies are in the ratio 2:1) have an essential similarity, and indeed are given the same name (C, D, etc.) in the traditional musical scale. It is also the case that other musical intervals correspond to simple ratios between the frequencies of the tones. For example, a fifth corresponds to a frequency ratio of 3:2, a major third to 5:4 and a minor third to 6:5. When musical notes in these simple ratios are sounded simultaneously, the sound is pleasant, or consonant, whereas departures from simple, integral, ratios, as in certain progressive modern music, tend to result in a less pleasant or even a dissonant sound. This does not always hold for pure tones, a pair of which tend to be judged as consonant as soon as their frequency separation exceeds a critical band (Plomp and Levelt, 1965). However, complex tones blend harmoniously and tend to produce chords only when their fundamental frequencies are in simple ratios. In this situation several of their harmonics will coincide, whereas for non-simple ratios the harmonics will differ in frequency, and produce beating sensations. Thus at least part of the dissonance may be explained in terms of this beating, or interference, of harmonics on the basilar membrane when the harmonics are close together, but not identical, in frequency. This cannot account for the whole of the effect, however; a pronounced dissonance from two mistuned pure tones may be heard when the tones are presented one to each ear. It is of interest, then, to consider why we prefer certain frequency ratios, for both the simultaneous and successive presentation of tones, why octaves sound so similar, and why some sounds are consonant and others dissonant.

One type of theory suggests that we learn about octave relationships and about other musical intervals by exposure to harmonic complex sounds (usually speech sounds) from the earliest moments in life. For example, the first two harmonics in a periodic sound will have a frequency ratio 2:1, the 2nd and 3rd will have a ratio 3:2, the 3rd and 4th 4:3, etc. Thus by exposure to these sounds we learn to associate harmonics with particular frequency ratios. We discussed earlier in this chapter Terhardt's (1972c) suggestion that such a learning process could account for the phenomenon of the perceptual 'stretching' of the octave. If judgements of similarity and of consonance or dissonance also depend upon familiarity, then a learning process will also account for our perception of other musical intervals (Terhardt, 1974).

An alternative theory suggests that we prefer pairs of tones for which there is a similarity in the time patterns of neural discharge. This view was put forward as early as 1898 by Mcyer, and has since been supported by Boomsliter and Creel (1961), among others. If it is the case that the pitch of a complex tone results from an analysis and correlation of the temporal patterns of firing in different groups of auditory neurones, then such an analysis would also reveal similarities between different tones when they are in simple frequency ratios. It is certainly the case that both our sense of musical pitch and our ability to make octave matches largely disappear above 5 kHz, the frequency at which neural synchrony no longer appears to operate. Furthermore, the highest note (fundamental) for instruments in the orchestra lies just below 5 kHz. One could argue from this that our lack of musical pitch at high frequencies is a result of a lack of exposure to tones at these frequencies. However, notes produced by musical instruments do contain harmonics above 5 kHz, so that if the learning of associations between harmonics were the only factor involved, there would be no reason for the change at 5 KHz.

It is of interest that the musical scale in general use today does not consist of notes in exact simple ratios. The common scale, the equal temperament (ET) scale, enables musicians to play in any key they choose, whereas with a system involving simple ratios only one key could be used. In the ET scale the octave (which still corresponds to a frequency ratio of 2:1) is divided into 12 equal logarithmic steps, known as semitones. Each successive semitone has a frequency about 5.9 per cent higher than its neighbour. The deviations from a simple ratio scale are small, although they are probably great enough to produce noticeable increases in the beating of harmonics of simultaneously presented complex tones at several points in the scale. While simple ratios may be preferable for simultaneously presented tones, it is not clear whether this is the case for tones presented successively. A number of experiments investigating preferred notes in performances on stringed instruments of various kinds have shown that there is no simple answer. Some workers have found preferences for simple ratios, while others have found that the preferred scale corresponds fairly closely to ET, except that notes higher than the tonic or key-note tend to be sharpened relative to that note. Boomsliter and Creel (1963) asked musicians to play familiar tunes on a monochord, a one-stringed instrument with continuously variable tuning. They found that while subjects consistently chose the same tuning for a given note within a given tune, they chose different tunings, for what is ostensibly the same note, in different melodies and in different parts of the same melody. However, Boomsliter and Creel found that the chosen patterns formed a structure of small whole number ratios to the tonic and to additional reference notes linked by small whole number ratios to the tonic. Thus within small groups of notes simple ratios are preferred, although the 'reference' point may vary as the melody proceeds.

Whether or not there is something inherently preferable about simple frequency ratios, it is clear that individual differences, cultural background, etc., can influence significantly the muscial combinations that are judged to be 'pleasant' or otherwise. Thus, for example,

Indian musical scales contain 'microtones' in which the conventional scale is subdivided into smaller units, producing many musical intervals which do not correspond to simple ratios. Indian music often sounds strange to western ears, especially on first hearing, but it clearly does not sound strange to Indians; indeed, the microtones, and the various different scales which can be composed from them, are held to add considerably to the richness of the music and to the variety of moods which it can create.

While there is a psychoacoustic basis for consonance and dissonance judgements, these judgements also display individual differences and follow changes in the cultural norm. Modern classical music, for example, by Stravinsky and Stockhausen, contains many examples of chords which would have been considered dissonant 20 years ago but which are now enjoyed by many people.

4.5.2 *Absolute pitch and tone deafness*

Some people have the ability to recognise and define the pitch of a musical tone without reference to a comparison tone. This faculty is called absolute pitch, and is quite rare, probably occurring in less than 1 per cent of the population. It seems to be distinct from the ability which some people develop to judge the pitch of a note in relation to, say, the lowest note which they can sing. Rakowski (1972) investigated absolute pitch by asking observers to adjust a variable signal so as to have the same pitch as a standard signal, for various time delays between the standard and variable tones. He used two groups of subjects, one group having been specially selected for their absolute pitch. For long time delays the subjects without absolute pitch showed a marked deterioration in performance, presumably because the pitch sensation stored in memory was lost. The subjects with absolute pitch seemed able to recall this memory with the aid of their 'imprinted' pitch standards, so that only a small decrement in performance was observed. And when the standard tone belonged to the normal musical scale (e.g. $A_2 = 110$ Hz) there was hardly any decrement in performance with increasing time delay. The subjects did not seem able to acquire new standards and never, for example, learned to remember a 1000 Hz tone 'as such'; it was always recalled as being a little lower than C_6. Attempts to improve absolute pitch identification by intensive training have met with some success (Cuddy, 1968), but the levels of performance achieved rarely equal those found in genuine cases of absolute pitch. It seems likely that absolute pitch is a faculty acquired through 'imprinting' in childhood a limited number of standards. Ward (1963a, b; 1970) has suggested that the converse is true; we may all start with a sense of absolute pitch, but the ability is trained out of us because we are reinforced for relative and not absolute pitch judgements. The limited success achieved by training in adulthood tends, at the moment, to favour the idea of some sort of imprinting.

The term 'tone deafness' is a misnomer, since nearly everyone is able to judge that two tones are different in pitch when their frequency difference exceeds a certain amount. Many people, on the other hand, have difficulty in reproducing (i.e. singing) musical notes or sequences of notes, often because the notes fall outside the normal range which they would produce in speaking. It is likely that practice effects, and musical experience in general, have a considerable influence on this ability. A second difficulty commonly experienced by naive listeners is that of assigning a direction to a pitch change; they can often hear that two tones are different, but they cannot decide which is the higher in pitch. These people show a considerable improvement with practice, and it is usually found that listeners who claim to be tone-deaf are eventually able to make very fine frequency discriminations. Beckett and Haggard (1973) did, however, find large differences in initial discrimination level between self-assessed musical and non-musical subjects, and it is of interest why such large differences arise. Very probably both genetic and environmental factors are involved.

There may be culture-bound differences in the ability to judge pitch changes. Tanner and Rivette (1964) tested three Indian subjects who had difficulty in judging the direction of frequency changes as large as 4 per cent. These observers cannot have been tone-deaf in a psychoacoustical sense, since their native language, Punjabi, contains a functional tone; this means that different pitches and pitch changes give words with different meanings as heard by the Punjabi listener, where we would hear the same word with a different pitch or pitch inflection. The difficulty of these subjects is probably related to some other factor, possibly that of assigning a direction to a pitch change, or possibly simply unfamiliarity with the non-linguistic task involved. The Tanner and Rivette finding underlines the need mentioned earlier not to attribute automatically to perceptual processes the patterns of performance we see in experimental results.

Pitch Perception

4.6 AUDITORY PATTERNS

Two common remarks about auditory psychophysics are that scant study has been made of pattern perception and that the time dimension has a special role in auditory experience. These remarks are not only true, but also connected. In general, the ability to identify one object from a large set of objects depends upon there being several dimensions along which the objects vary. Our ability to make an absolute identification of stimuli varying along a single dimension (e.g. pitch) begins to break down when the number of stimuli exceeds about 5–6 (Pollack, 1952). It is in this respect that the time dimension is crucial in hearing, since in hearing there is only one dimension mapping into neural place in a way that is both straightforward and precise, namely frequency. In order to identify auditory 'objects' more dimensions are required (although, as we shall see in a moment, the frequency dimension may itself be regarded as multidimensional). Auditory space does not provide the extra dimensions required, because it defines where, rather than what, an object is. Thus auditory pattern or 'object' perception has to depend on structures in frequency and in time, of which music and speech represent advanced forms.

Consider first time-invariant patterns. If a single frequency is presented, then the pattern can be described by just two numbers, specifying frequency and intensity. However, almost all of the sounds which we encounter in everyday life are considerably more complex than this, and contain a multitude of frequencies at many different intensity levels. Thus psychologists have sought ways of describing the frequency spectrum so that the information content is psychologically realistic. This has been attempted both for speech and for non-speech sounds by Plomp and his colleagues (Plomp, Pols and van de Geer, 1967; Plomp, 1970), using a technique which differs only slightly from factor analysis and other standard ways of reducing the dimensionality of the variable data obtained in the biological sciences. Firstly, a spectrum is characterised with a set of numbers representing the amplitudes in some 18 one-third octave frequency bands. This relatively broad-band analysis achieves a basic economy consistent with the frequency-analysing power of the peripheral auditory system; critical bands are roughly one-third octave in width over a fairly wide frequency range. A representative sample of spectra is then obtained (e.g. the vowels of a language spoken by a set of speakers with subjectively different voices). The level in each one-third octave band will vary as a function of vowel or speaker, but the levels in different bands will not be entirely independent, particularly for bands of adjacent frequency. Thus the information about the vowel or speaker conveyed by the levels in the 18 one-third octave bands is redundant, or partially duplicated. This redundancy can be eliminated by statistical procedures that yield the chief higher-order dimensions underlying the differences between sounds in the sample chosen. Each higher-order dimension will be a weighted function of each of the original 18 amplitude dimensions. Different sets of higher-order dimensions will be obtained according to whether we emphasise the differences between different vowels or the differences between different speakers.

This procedure results in a reduction in the number of dimensions needed to account for the differences between the different spectra in the set. In general, the more the number of dimensions is reduced, the less well is it possible to account for these differences. Three dimensions are sufficient to account for about 82 per cent of the total variation. Thus, with a reasonably small error, each vowel can be represented as a point in a three-dimensional space. If we take into account variations between different speakers, or between the same speaker on different occasions, the representation of each vowel becomes a 'blob' or a certain volume in this three-dimensional space.

Consider now the subjective significance of these higher-order dimensions. To investigate this Pols, van der Kamp and Plomp (1969) also carried out perceptual analyses of their vowel stimuli, using a technique based on triadic comparison. In this method the subject has to decide, for each possible subset of three stimuli, which pair is most similar and which pair is least similar. On the dasis of these judgements a multidimensional perceptual space can be constructed for the different vowel sounds. (The exact method by which this is done is rather complex. The interested reader is referred to Shepard, 1962, and Kruskal, 1964.) Each vowel is represented as a point in the multidimensional space, and the greater the distance between these points the more dissimilar are the vowels judged to be. As was the case for the physical analysis, the number of dimensions can be reduced at the expense of a loss of 'goodness of fit'. When Pols and co-workers compared the three-dimensional physical configuration with the three-dimensional perceptual configuration, they found a close correspondence; the correlation coefficients for the three dimensions were 0.992, 0.971 and 0.742. When six dimensions were used, the correlation coefficients were even higher. Pols and co-workers summed up these results as follows: 'From this remarkable correspondence, it can be concluded that the subjects used for their perceptual judgements information comparable with that present in the physical representation of these signals. The perceptual differences between the stimuli, to be considered as timbre differences, appear to be qualified by their differences in frequency spectra.'

It should not be assumed that the dimensions derived by Pols and co-workers represent *the* chief mode of functioning of a *fixed* set of pattern analysers, or that the number of dimensions involved in timbre judgements is necessarily small. It is likely that the number of dimensions required is limited by the number of critical bands required to cover the audible frequency range. This would give a maximum of 23 dimensions, or, if we exclude very high and very low frequencies, about 15. For a restricted class of sounds, however, a much smaller set of dimensions may be involved.

Although differences in static timbre may enable us to distinguish between two sounds presented successively, they are not always sufficient to allow the absolute identification of an 'auditory object', such as a musical instrument. One reason for this is that the frequency spectrum may be strongly altered by the transmission path of the sound. In practice recognition may depend upon a number of different factors (see those suggested by Schouten, which we described at the beginning of this chapter), but, in particular, on onset transients and on the envelopes of the sounds. For example, the characteristic tone of a piano depends on the fact that the notes are decaying. If a recording of a piano is reversed in time, the timbre is completely different. It now resembles that of a harmonium or accordion, in spite of the fact that the harmonic content is unchanged. Thus rapid changes in loudness or harmonic structure may be crucial for the identification of an instrument. In addition, many instruments have noise-like qualities which strongly influence their subjective quality. A flute, for example, has a relatively simple harmonic structure, but synthetic tones with the same harmonic structure do not sound flute-like unless each note is preceded by a small 'puff' of noise. In general, tones of standard musical instruments are poorly simulated by the summation of steady component frequencies (this is what an electronic organ usually does), since such a synthesis cannot produce the dynamic variation with time characteristic of these instruments.

4.6.1 *Temporal patterning*

Just as sounds can be patterned according to the amount of energy in different frequency regions, so also can they be patterned according to how they vary as a function of time. Many of the auditory sequences occurring naturally are rhythmic, so that one might reasonably expect that the perceptual mechanisms are designed to make use of these rhythms (Sturges and Martin, 1974). If an auditory pattern is rhythmic, then certain elements in the pattern are temporarily redundant, so that once early elements of the pattern are heard, later elements, and possibly the end of the pattern as well, can be anticipated.

A number of workers have investigated the 'perceptual organisation' or subjective grouping of repeating sequences of two elements (e.g. a high-pitched buzz and a low-pitched buzz). Royer and Garner (1966, 1970) found that subjects usually organised the pattern beginning at specific elements (subjects were required to give verbal reports of the way the sequences were perceived). These elements, termed preferred start points, either began a run of identical elements or were chosen to produce a pattern ending in a run of identical elements (HHHLHLHL or LHLHLHHH). If the temporal patterns were made more complex by the addition of features such as temporal pauses or intensity accents, organisation could be either by these features or by the pattern structure of the elements. If pattern structure was made to conflict with the pause organisation, by inserting a temporal pause before a non-preferred start point (HHLHLHLH HHLHLHLH...), the pause organisation was dominant. These experiments indicate a powerful subjective tendency for such patterns to be perceived as organised wholes, with the physical characteristics which determine the organisation being arranged in a hierarchical manner. Handel (1973) has confirmed that if repeating patterns are segmented by temporal pauses, the pattern perception is based on the structure of the temporal grouping rather than by the structure of the pattern elements. In other words, the exact timing of the elements is more important in determining the subjective rhythm than is the patterning of the elements themselves (produced by pitch variations in this case).

In all the experiments on temporal patterning that we have described so far, the rate of presentation of elements was relatively slow (3–4 elements per second), and all the elements in the pattern were perceived as being part of a single pattern. When we listen to fast tone sequences (say ten per second), this does not always happen. The tones are not grouped simply according to their physical temporal order, but according to their attributes, e.g. their pitches. This has been called rhythmic fission. van Noorden (1971) investigated this phenomenon using a tone sequence where every second B was omitted from the regular sequence ABABAB . . ., producing a sequence ABA ABA . . . He found that this could be perceived in two ways, depending on the frequency separation of A and B. For small separations a single rhythm, resembling a gallop, is heard. For larger separations two separate tone sequences can be heard, one of which is running twice as fast as the other. van Noorden found that it was possible to establish two different boundaries between fusion and fission, according to the instructions given and the set of the subject. The inner boundary, within which fusion always occurs, depends primarily on the frequency separation of the two tones, and varies according to centre frequency. The outer boundary depends also upon the silent interval between successive tone pulses. For time intervals less than 100 ms fission will nearly always occur provided that the frequencies of the tones are separated by more than about 20–30 per cent. For silent intervals longer than 100 ms there is a much wider range of frequency separations over which either fusion or fission may occur, depending on the set of the subject. It may be that subjects are only able to switch attention between different frequency bands, in order to achieve fusion, at a limited rate of about one octave per 100 ms.

Dowling (1968) has shown that rhythmic fission may also occur when successive tones differ in intensity or in spatial location. Thus the perceptual organisation of a rhythmic sound may depend on a number of physical characteristics of that sound. Dowling found that embedding a melody in alternate tones of the same intensity and randomly selected from the same frequency range produced a meaningless jumble. Making the tune different, either in frequency range or in spatial location, enabled subjects to pick it out. It seems likely that timbre differences may also contribute to rhythmic fission, since in a piece of polyphonic music with interwoven themes played on different instruments we are able to pick out the separate themes even when the instruments are coming from the same direction (e.g. via a loudspeaker) and are playing notes in the same frequency range.

A number of composers have exploited the fact that rhythmic fission occurs for tones widely separated in frequency. By playing a sequence of tones in which alternate notes are chosen from separate frequency ranges, an instrument such as the flute, which is only capable of playing one note at a time, can appear to be playing two themes at once. Many fine examples of this are available in the works of Bach. Laboratory studies investigating this effect have been reported by Dowling (1973).

A phenomenon which is probably related to that of rhythmic fission occurs in judgements of the temporal order of sounds. Ladefoged and Broadbent (1960) reported that extraneous sounds in sentences were grossly mislocalised, so that a click might be reported as occurring a word or two away from its actual position. Surprisingly poor performance was also reported by Warren *et al.* (1969), for judgements of the temporal order of three or four unrelated items, such as a hiss, a tone and a buzz. Most subjects could not identify the order when successive items lasted as long as 200 ms, and naïve subjects required component durations of at least 700 ms to perceive the order of four sounds presented in an uninterrupted series of repeated sequences. These durations are well above those which are normally considered necessary for temporal resolution in speech and music. (Winckel, 1967, reported that the temporal order of musical notes is resolvable down to about 50 ms per note.) Further, it is known that for smaller numbers of items the threshold duration for discrimination is much smaller; Hirsh (1959) found that for pairs of unrelated items durations as small as 20 ms still allowed correct order discrimination.

There are a number of ways of viewing the poor order discrimination described by Warren *et al.* The sounds they used do not represent a coherent class, although they are all non-speech. They have different waveform and spectral characteristics, and, as for tones widely differing in frequency, they do not form a single auditory stream. As a consequence, they float about with respect to each other in subjective time, in much the same way as a click superimposed on speech. Further, since one sound changes abruptly into another, there are no transitional cues, such as changes in frequency, which could be detected as such and used to define unambiguously the temporal order. It should be emphasised that the relatively poor performance reported by Warren *et al.* is found only in tasks requiring absolute identification of the order of sounds, and not in tasks which simply require the discrimination of different sequences. Further, with extended training and feedback subjects can be trained to distinguish between *and* identify orders within sequences of non-related sounds lasting only 10 ms or less (Warren, 1974). For sequences of tones the component duration necessary for correct order identification may be as low as 2–7 ms (Divenyi and Hirsh, 1974). To explain these effects Divenyi and Hirsh suggested that two kinds of perceptual judgements are involved. At longer component durations the listener is able to hear a clear sequence of steady state sounds, whereas at shorter durations a change in the order of components introduces qualitative changes that are capable of being discriminated by the trained listener. Similar explanations have been put forward by Green (1973) and Warren (1974).

Bregman and Campbell (1971) investigated the factors that make temporal order judgements for tone sequences difficult. They used naïve subjects, so that performance presumably depended on the subjects actually perceiving the sounds as a sequence, rather than on them learning the overall sound pattern. They found that in a repeating cycle of mixed high and low tones subjects could discriminate the order of the high tones relative to one another, or of the low tones among themselves, but they could not order the high tones relative to the low ones. The authors suggested that this was because the two groups of sounds split into separate perceptual streams, a process they called 'primary auditory stream, segregation', and that judgements across streams are difficult. In a further investigation of this effect Bregman and Dannenbring (1973) used tone sequences in which successive tones were connected by frequency glides. They found that these glides reduced the tendency for the sequences to split into high and low streams, while at the same time order perception was easier. Conditions using partial glides also showed decreased stream segregation, although the partial glides were not quite as effective as complete glides. Thus complete continuity between tones is not required to reduce stream segregation; a frequency change 'pointing' towards the next tone allows the listener to follow the pattern more easily.

The effects of frequency glides, and other types of transitions, in preventing stream segregation or fission are probably of considerable importance in the perception of speech. Speech sounds may follow one another in very rapid sequences, so that the glides and partial glides observed in the acoustic components of speech may be a strong factor in maintaining the speech as a unified stream. Experimental evidence in favour of this idea has been presented by Cole and Scott (1974). Their work, and other relevant work, will be discussed more fully in Chapter 6.

Another way in which the streaming phenomenon is relevant to speech perception is illustrated by studies using synthetic speech. In such large fluctuations of an unexpected kind in the fundamental frequency give the impression that a new speaker has stepped in to take over a few syllables from the primary one. Although a single speaker's fundamental frequencies do cover a range of about one octave, the intrusion effect is observed with smaller jumps than this, provided they are inconsistent with the changes in the fundamental required by the linguistic and phonetic context. Thus it appears that the assignment of incoming spectral patterns to particular speakers is done on the basis of fundamental frequency, but in a predictive manner; only deviations from the anticipated fundamental are interpreted as a new speaker.

4.7 GENERAL CONCLUSIONS

We have discussed in this chapter how the perception of pitch and timbre is related to the physical properties of the stimuli and to the anatomical and physiological properties of the auditory system. In principle, there are two ways in which the frequency of a sound may be coded: by the temporal patterns of firing in auditory neurones and by the distribution of excitation among different fibres. It is likely that both types of information are utilised but that their relative importance is different for different frequency ranges and different types of signals.

The neurophysiological evidence in animals indicates that synchrony of nerve impulses to a particular phase of the stimulating waveform disappears above 4–5 kHz. Above this frequency our ability to discriminate changes in the frequency of pure tones diminishes, and our sense of musical pitch disappears. It is likely that this reflects our use of temporal information in the frequency range below 4–5 kHz.

For complex tones the pitch may be derived by a mechanism operating on the neural signals corresponding to individual partials in the complex, or it may be coded in the time pattern of neural impulses derived from a point on the basilar membrane where partials are interfering. The former mechanism, which is a sort of pattern recogniser, will tend to operate when stimuli contain low harmonics or contain only a small number of harmonics, whereas the latter mechanism will operate when only high harmonics are present. For both types of mechanism, combination tones in the frequency region below the lowest presented partial may influence the pitch percept.

It is not yet clear whether the 'pattern recogniser' derives the pitch of a complex tone from the spatial distribution of activity in different nerve fibres or from the time patterns of neural activity in different fibres. However, residue pitches are only perceived when partials or combination tones are present in the frequency range where temporal information would be available. Thus a mechanism which operates by comparing or correlating the results of an analysis of the time patterns of firing in different channels seems the most plausible. Such a mechanism could account for our ability to assign harmonics to the appropriate fundamental when we listen to two complex tones simultaneously.

For complex tones phenomena involving periodicity mechanisms (e.g. the missing fundamental) are only observed for fundamental frequencies below about 1400 Hz, whereas for pure tones the upper limit for the operation of temporal mechanisms probably lies around 4–5 kHz. In the past the upper limit of 1400 Hz observed for complex tones has been assumed to apply to temporal mechanisms in general, including those relating to pure tones. There is, however, no need to make this assumption; indeed, there are good reasons for expecting different upper limits for pure tones and complex tones. Periodicity phenomena for complex tones can only be observed when harmonics above the 2nd are present. In general, harmonics around the 3rd, 4th and 5th will dominate the pitch percept, if they are present. If we also require that these harmonics lie in the region where temporal mechanisms are operating (i.e. below 4–5 kHz), it is clear that the upper limit for the observation of periodicity phenomena for complex tones will lie below this by a factor of about 3, i.e. about 1400 Hz.

Certain aspects of the perception of music may be related to basic mechanisms underlying pitch perception. There is some evidence, for example, that we prefer musical intervals, or pairs of tones, for which there is a similarity in the time patterns of neural discharge. On the other hand, it is clear that early experience, individual differences, cultural background, etc., also play a significant role in such judgements. Whether these latter variables in turn influence the basic mechanisms is likely to remain unclear for many years, until appropriately controlled cross-cultural and developmental studies can be done.

The perception of auditory patterns depends upon variations in both frequency spectrum and time. For static spectra, and a restricted class of sounds, a limited number of dimensions may be sufficient to describe variations in the sounds. The subjective organisation of temporal sequences of sounds depends upon the physical characteristics of the sounds and upon their exact timing. Judgements of temporal order depend uppn the frequency differences between elements, and may be strongly affected by perceptual 'stream segregation'. The reduction in stream segregation produced by frequency glides may be of considerable importance in the perception of speech.

5

Space Perception

5.1 INTRODUCTION

The ability to localise sound sources is of considerable importance to both humans and animals; it will determine the direction of objects to seek or to avoid, as well as indicating the appropriate direction to direct visual attention. The precision of sound localisation is remarkable, particularly for brief sounds, or for those occurring in noisy or reverberant surroundings. While the most reliable cues used in the localisation of sounds depend upon a comparison of the signals reaching the two ears, there are also phenomena of auditory space perception which result from monaural processing of the signals.

The term 'localisation' refers to judgements of the direction and distance of a sound source. Sometimes, when headphones are worn, the sound image is located inside the head. The term 'lateralisation' is used to describe the apparent location of the sound source within the head. Headphones allow precise control of interaural differences and eliminate effects related to room echos. Thus lateralisation may be regarded as a laboratory version of localisation which provides an efficient means of studying direction perception.

While our binaural abilities are important for the accurate location of sounds, this is not their only function. Using two ears, we are able to selectively attend to sounds coming from a particular direction while effectively excluding other sounds. This ability is particularly important in noisy surroundings, or when there are several sound sources competing for our attention. Laboratory studies of this phenomenon have shown that the conditions which produce the most well-defined spatial separations of 'signal' and 'noise' do not necessarily produce the best detection performance.

Thus, while the 'cocktail-party' phenomenon is probably closely related to our ability to locate sounds in space, the underlying processes may be different (see Section 5.8.1).

As well as being able to judge the direction of a sound source, we are able, in some cases, to estimate its distance. This ability is particularly developed in blind people, who can use information from echoes and reflections to determine the positions of objects in the environment.

5.2 THE LOCALISATION OF PURE TONES AND BINAURAL BEATS

The cues which enable us to localise sounds may vary depending on the nature of those sounds. We consider first steady sinusoidal sounds. Later on we discuss a much more common class of sounds: those which are discontinuous, or contain transients.

Consider a sinusoidal sound source lying to one side of the head. The sound reaching the farther ear will be delayed in time and will be less intense relative to the nearer ear. There are thus two possible cues as to the location of the sound source. However, owing to the physical nature of the sounds, these cues are not equally effective at all frequencies. Low-frequency sounds have a wavelength which is long compared with the size of the head, and thus the sound 'bends' very well around the head. This process is known as diffraction, and the result is that little or no 'shadow' is cast by the head. On the other hand, at high frequencies, where the wavelength is short compared with the dimensions of the head, little diffraction occurs. A 'shadow' almost like that produced by a beam of light, occurs. Interaural differences in intensity are negligible at low frequencies, but may be as large as 20 dB at high frequencies. This may easily be illustrated by placing a small transistor radio close to one ear. If that ear is now blocked with a finger, only sound bending around the head and entering the other ear will be heard. The sound will be much less 'tinny', since high frequencies will have been attenuated more than low; the head effectively acts like a low-pass filter. Interaural intensity differences will thus be more important at high frequencies than at low.

If a tone is delayed in one ear relative to the other, then there will be a phase difference between the two ears; thus, if nerve impulses occur at a particular phase of the stimulating waveform, the rela-

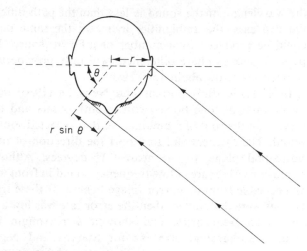

Figure 5.1 Illustrating the difference in arrival time at the two ears for a distant sound source at an angle θ radians to the observer. If we denote the radius of the head (about 3.5 in or 9 cm) by r, then the path difference d between the two ears is given by

$$d = r\theta + r\sin\theta.$$

For a sound directly to one side of the observer $\theta = \pi/2$ radians and $d = (3.5 \times \pi/2) + (3.5 \times \sin \pi/2) = 9$ in (23 cm). Since sound takes about 76 μs to travel 1 in, the corresponding time delay is about 680 μs.

tive timing of the nerve impulses at the two ears will be related to the location of the sound source. However, for sounds whose wavelength is comparable with, or less than, the distance between the two ears there will be ambiguity. The maximum path difference between the two ears is about 9 in (23 cm), which corresponds to a time delay of about 680 μs (see Figure 5.1). Ambiguities will first occur when the half-wavelength of the sound is about 9 in, i.e. when the frequency of the sound is about 750 Hz. At this point a sound lying to one side of the head will produce waveforms at the two ears which are in opposite phase (phase difference between the two ears of 180 degrees). From the observer's point of view the location of the sound source is now ambiguous, since the waveform at the right ear might be either a half-cycle behind that at the left ear or a half-cycle ahead. Head movements, or movements of the sound source, may resolve this ambiguity, so that there will be no abrupt upper limit in our ability to use phase differences between the two ears. However, when the wavelength of the sound is less than the path difference between the two ears, the ambiguities increase; the same phase difference could be produced by a number of different source locations. For periodic sounds phase differences will only provide useful cues for frequencies below about 1500 Hz.

In a classic study Stevens and Newman (1936) investigated the localisation of tone bursts with smooth onsets and offsets for observers on the roof of a building, so that reflected sounds were minimised. The listeners had to report the direction of the source, in a horizontal plane, to the nearest 15 degrees. Although left–right confusions were rare, a low-frequency sound in front was often indistinguishable from its mirror image behind. If these front–back confusions were discounted, then the error rate was low at very low and very high frequencies, and showed a maximum for mid-range frequencies (around 3000 Hz for Stevens and Newman's data). These data were taken to indicate two different mechanisms for sound localisation, one operating best at high frequencies and one at low. For middle frequencies neither mechanism operates efficiently, and errors are at a maximum.

These results have been broadly confirmed by more recent experiments (Sandel *et al.*, 1955) using anechoic chambers, except that systematic biases have been found in addition to errors; there is a tendency to underestimate the deviation of the source from the median plane when the frequency of the tone is between 1500 and 5000 Hz. When these systematic errors are eliminated, the greatest uncertainty in localisation occurs at a frequency of about 1500 Hz. Sandel *et al.* also used an arrangement of two loudspeakers such that the resultant combined tone led in phase at one ear, but had a greater amplitude in the other. They found that the sound was located towards the side with the phase lead for frequencies below about 1500 Hz and towards the side with greater amplitude for frequencies above this. Near 1500 Hz listeners were confused.

These experiments confirm that the extent to which the cues of interaural time and intensity differences are used in the localisation of pure tones is strongly related to what would be predicted from the physical nature of these cues. Intensity differences are more important at high frequencies, while phase differences only provided usable cues for frequencies below about 1500 Hz. Experiments using headphones (Mills, 1960) have shown that we are able to detect differences in intensity at the two ears even for low frequencies and that these differences can produce a sense of location to one side. The smallest detectable change for low frequencies is, however, larger than would occur in real life except under exceptional circumstances (e.g. holding a telephone close to one ear).

A phenomenon which seems to be closely related to the ability of the auditory system to process phase differences at the two ears is that of binaural beats. These may occur when a tone of one frequency is presented to one ear and a tone of slightly differing frequency is presented to the other ear. The sound appears to fluctuate or warble at a rate corresponding to the frequency difference between the two tones. Notice that binaural beats are quite different from the physical beats which are produced when the two frequencies are mixed in the electrical or acoustical system. Such physical beats or 'uniaural' beats occur because the two frequencies are alternately in phase and out of phase, and thus alternately cancel and reinforce one another; the intensity fluctuates at a rate depending on the frequency difference between the two tones. Binaural beats, on the other hand, depend upon an interaction in the nervous system of the inputs from the two ears, and have been considered to provide a demonstration that the discharges of neurones in the auditory nerve preserve information about the phase of the acoustic stimulus. If neural firings tend to occur at a particular phase of the stimulating waveform, then at some common neural centre the trains of neural firings from the two ears will superimpose differently depending on the relative phase of the stimuli at the two ears. There is thus a nerual basis for the subjective fluctuations which occur when the relative phase at the two cars fluctuates as it does when tones with slightly different frequencies are presented to the two ears.

Since binaural beats differ in their origin from 'uniaural' beats, it is hardly surprising that the two kinds of beats differ subjectively; binaural beats are never as distinct as uniaural beats. In addition, Licklider, Webster and Hedlun (1950) pointed out that there is a continuum of subjective effects depending on the frequency separation of the two tones. As the frequency separation is slowly increased from zero, the listener may hear a tone that periodically shifts in subjective location, then fluctuates in loudness, then seems 'rough' and finally separates into two subjectively smooth tones. Uniaural beats can be observed over the entire audible frequency range, whereas binaural beats are essentially a low-frequency phenomenon. Estimates of the highest frequency for which binaural beats can be observed have varied. The beats are heard most distinctly for frequencies between 300 and 600 Hz, but become progressively more difficult to hear at high frequencies. The exact upper limit depends upon the intensity used and upon the experimental technique, but it is generally agreed that the beats are exceedingly difficult to hear for frequencies above 1000 Hz (Licklider *et al.*, 1950). Uniaural beats are most distinctly heard when the two tones are matched for intensity, and cannot be heard at all when the intensities of the two tones differ greatly. Binaural beats, however, can be heard when there are large differences in intensity at the two ears (Tobias, 1963), and may even be heard when the tone to one ear is below absolute threshold (Groen, 1964). Thus phase-locking seems to occur over a wide range of stimulus intensities.

One interesting feature of binaural beats is that the upper limit of the frequency at which they are perceived is higher for men than for women. Further, the upper limit for women changes with the menstrual cycle, so that just at the onset of menstrual flow the upper limit for women approaches that of men (Tobias, 1965; Haggard and Bates, 1974). These changes are presumably related to hormonal variations and variations in retained body fluid, both of which could affect nerve transmission. It is possible that similar variations in performance will be observed for other kinds of tasks which are influenced by the timing of nerve impulses, e.g. the localisation of sounds and the perception of residue pitches. Indeed, the extent to which such variations occur could be used to assess the importance of temporal information in these tasks.

5.3 THE IMPORTANCE OF TRANSIENTS

All sounds which occur in nature have onsets and offsets, and many also change their intensity or their spectral structure as a function of time. Interaural differences in the time of arrival of these transients provide cues for the localisation of these sounds which are not subject to the phase ambiguities which occur for steady tones. Such cues are often eliminated in experiments using pure tones, by turning the tones on and off very slowly, although for pure tones the transient cues may be comparable in effectiveness to the continuously available cues of ongoing intensity and phase differences. Klump and Eady (1956) measured thresholds for the detection of interaural time differences using stimuli delivered via headphones. They compared three types of stimuli: band-limited noise (containing frequencies in the range 150–1700 Hz), 1000 Hz pure tones with gradual rise and fall times, and clicks of duration 1 ms. The first stimulus varies continuously as a function of time, and thus provides transient information which is repeated many times during the presentation time of the stimulus; the pure tone provides only information relating to ongoing phase differences; while the click is effectively a single transient. The threshold interaural time differences were 9 μs, 11 μs and 28 μs. Thus the greatest acuity occurred for the noise stimulus, with continuously available transient information, but the tone gave performance which was only slightly worse. The single click gave rise to the poorest performance. It is worth noting, however, that the tones in this experiment were of relatively long duration (1.4 s). For tones of shorter duration our acuity is not so great, so that cues related to onset and offset transients (which would be comparable to those provided by the clicks) become relatively more important.

For sounds with ongoing transient disparities, such as bursts of noise, our ability to detect interaural time differences improves with duration of the bursts for durations up to about 700 ms, when the threshold disparity (the smallest detectable time difference at the two ears) reaches an asymptotic level of about 6 μs (Tobias and Zerlin, 1959). It is remarkable that such small time differences between the ears are detectable, since the average synaptic latency is about 1000 μs, with a variability of perhaps 500 μs. Tobias (1972) has discussed some of the ways in which this accuracy might be achieved, including the possibility that there is a direct neural pathway from one cochlea to the other. At the present time, however, the neural mechanism by which we discriminate these remarkably small time intervals remains a mystery.

Tobias and Schubert (1959) investigated the relative importance of onset disparities and ongoing disparities in lateralisation judgements by pitting one against the other. They presented bursts of noise via headphones, with a particular onset time difference, and determined the amount of ongoing disparity needed to counteract the onset information and recentre the subjective image. They found that small ongoing disparities offset much larger transient onset disparities and that for durations exceeding 300 ms the onset has no effect. Even for short bursts (10 ms) the ongoing disparity has the greater effect. For very short impulsive sounds the importance of onset disparity will be much greater; for brief clicks this will be the only kind of transient disparity. It is worth noting that for high-frequency pure tones the ongoing phase differences at the two ears are not processed by the auditory system. However, these tones can still be lateralised on the basis of onset transient disparities.

Stimuli such as noises and clicks contain energy over a wide range of frequencies. Yost, Wightman and Green (1971) attempted to determine which frequency components were the most important, by studying the lateralisation of clicks whose frequency content had been altered by filtering. The subjects were asked to discriminate a centred image (produced by identical clicks at each ear) from a displaced image (produced by delaying the click to the left ear only). They found that discrimination deteriorated for clicks which were high-pass filtered, so that only energy above 1500 Hz was present, but was largely unaffected by low-pass filtering. Masking with a low-pass noise produced a marked disruption, while a high-pass noise had little effect. Thus it seems that the discrimination of lateral position on the basis of time delays between the two ears depends largely on the low-frequency content of the clicks, although some-what poorer discrimination is possible with only high-frequency components. This result is somewhat surprising at first sight, since the high-frequency components in the click contribute to the 'sharp-ness' of its edges (a low-pass filtered click will have longer rise and decay times) and therefore to the precision with which its timing can be defined. However, the finding ties in rather well with the results obtained with pure tones, showing that we cannot compare phases between the two ears for frequencies above 1500 Hz. When a click is presented to the ear, it produces a waveform, at a given point on the basilar mambrane, looking rather like a decaying sinusoidal oscillation (see Figure 1.10). The frequency of the oscillation will depend on which part of the basilar membrane is being observed; at the basal end the frequency will be high and at the apical end it will be low. For frequencies below 1500 Hz the phases of these decaying oscillations at the two ears can be compared, thus con-veying accurate information about the relative timing of the clicks at the two ears. For frequencies above 1500 Hz this 'fine structure' information will be lost; only timing information relating to the envelope of the decaying oscillation will be available at the point of binaural interaction, thus reducing the accuracy with which the clicks can be localised. (See Section 5.6 for further discussion on this point.)

Henning (1974) has provided further evidence for the importance of the amplitude envelope. He investigated the lateralisation of high-frequency tones which had been amplitude-modulated. (See Figure 3.4 for an illustration of this waveform.) He found that the detectability of interaural delays in the envelope of a 3900 Hz carrier modulated at a frequency of 300 Hz was about as good as the detectability of interaural delays in a 300 Hz pure tone. However, there were considerable differences among individual observers; the interaural delays necessary for 75 per cent correct detections in his forced-choice task had values of 20, 50 and 65 μs for three different subjects (all stimuli had 250 ms durations and 50 ms rise–fall times). Henning found that time delay of the envelope rather than time delay of the 'fine-structure' within the envelope determines the lateralisation. The signals could be lateralised on the basis of time delays in the envelope even when the carrier frequencies were different in the two ears. Thus it seems that for complex signals containing only high-frequency components, listeners extract the envelopes of the signals and compare the relative timing of the envelopes at the two ears. However, lateralisation performance is best when the carrier frequencies are identical, and poor lateralisation results when the complex waveforms at each ear have no frequency component in common. Thus factors other than the amplitude envelope can affect lateralisation performance.

At first sight there appears to be a discrepancy between the results of Henning and the results of Yost *et al.* (1971); Yost *et al.* found extremely poor lateralisation for clicks which had been filtered so as to contain only high-frequency components, whereas Henning found relatively good performance for AM tones containing only high-frequency components. The crucial difference is one of duration; in Henning's experiment many fluctuations in envelope amplitude occurred during the presentation time of the stimuli, while Yost *et al.* presented only single clicks. When Yost *et al.* presented a train of clicks, they found that performance for high-pass clicks improved with increasing duration. As Henning points out, these results indicate that duration is an important determinant of the detectability of interaural time differences.

It is worth noting that all the experiments described in this section were carried out using headphones. While this does not in any way negate the results, it does mean that cues related to interaural intensity differences have been eliminated. These cues may, in a normal

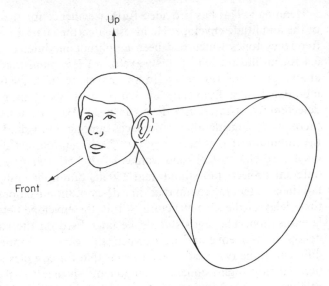

Figure 5.2 A cone of confusion for a spherical head and a particular interaural time delay. All sound sources on the surface of the cone would produce that interaural time delay. For details of how to calculate the cone of confusion see Mills (1972).

listening environment, have a significant effect on the localisation of sounds containing high-frequency components. Subjective impressions indicate that sounds containing high-frequency components may be easily and accurately located, and at least a part of this ease will be related to the intensity differences at the two ears and to the differences in spectral composition at the two ears which are produced by the low-pass action of the head and by the pinnae (see Section 5.4).

If we ignore, for the moment, the influence of the pinnae, then we may regard the head as a pair of holes separated by a spherical obstacle. If the head is kept stationary, then a given interaural time difference will not be sufficient uniquely to define the position of the sound source in space; there is a cone of confusion (see Mills, 1972, and Figure 5.2). The particular way that the ears are situated on the head also gives rise to the fact that we are much better at localising sounds in the horizontal dimension than in the vertical dimension. Ambiguities related to the cone of confusion, or to the location of a sound source in the vertical direction, may be resolved by head movements. If we rotate our heads about a vertical axis by, say, 20 degrees, and this results in a 20 degree shift in the apparent lateral position of the auditory image in relation to the head, then we locate the sound source in the horizontal plane. If the rotation of the head is accompanied by no change in the auditory image, then the sound is located either directly above or directly below the observer. Intermediate shifts in the location of the auditory image lead to intermediate vertical height judgements (Wallach, 1940). Hirsh (1971) has reviewed a number of experiments showing improved localisation abilities when head movements are allowed, so that in many cases monaural hearing is as good as binaural hearing (see below for further details). These experiments, and the results of a number of clinical studies, indicate that for hearing-aid wearers the ability to localise will be greater for head-worn aids than for body-worn aids (see below for further discussion of this point).

5.4 MONAURAL LOCALISATION AND THE ROLE OF THE PINNAE

A number of workers have reported that under some conditions the localisation of sounds with one ear can be as accurate as that with two, particularly if head movements are allowed (e.g. Freedman and Fisher, 1968). However, most of the experiments on monaural localisation have used rather coarse steps in degrees from one sound source (usually a loudspeaker) to the next, so that in many conditions nearly perfect performance was achieved for both monaural and binaural modes; in other words, the coarseness of the measure may well have obscured any superiority in binaural conditions. To overcome these problems, Harris and Sergeant (1971) instructed subjects to keep their heads as still as possible, and determined the Minimum Audible Angle (the smallest detectable change in angular position in the lateral plane, denoted MAA) for a moving sound source. The subjects listened (1) with both ears open, (2) with one ear plugged, muffed and noise-masked. They found that the monaural MAA was as small as the binaural MAA for white noise, but that for tones the monaural MAA was usually larger by a factor of 2 or more. For complex sounds, such as white noise, movements of either the head or the sound source produce changes in the spectral patterning at each ear (see below), and these changes provide cues as to the extent and direction of the movement. Thus for such complex sounds monaural localisation can be as good as binaural. For simple stimuli, such as pure tones, the binaural mode is superior, although moderately good localisation is still possible in the monaural mode.

While head movements, or movements of the sound source, are clearly important and can help to resolve ambiguities in vertical direction, our abilities at judging vertical direction are far in excess of what would be predicted if only information related to head movements or interaural differences were available. For example, we are able to judge the location of a burst of white noise in the median plane (the locus of points equidistant from the two ears) when the duration of the burst is too short to allow useful information to be gained from head movements.

Many workers have suggested that the action of the pinnae provides for verticality judgements (e.g. Butler, 1969) and for the discrimination of front from back, while others (e.g. Batteau, 1967; Freedman and Fisher, 1968) have suggested that the pinnae are important for localisation in every direction. Batteau investigated the action of the pinna using a scaled-up model, with a microphone inserted in the 'ear canal'. He found that the pinna transformed the incoming signal so that the initial signal was followed by a series of time-delayed replications. This kind of effect is limited to signals containing high-frequency components; only for frequencies above about 6 kHz is the wavelength of the sound sufficiently short to produce strong interactions with the pinna. For these high frequencies the sound enters the ear via a number of different paths: a direct path producing the initial signal, and several paths via the 'corrugations' in the pinna, producing the delayed replications. For lower frequencies the 'corrugations' have a negligible effect on the incoming sound. Batteau suggested that the pattern of delays differed characteristically according to locale, so that the encoding action of the pinna would in principle allow for a unique direction to be assigned to a sound source.

To investigate whether we are actually able to use these time delays, Batteau inserted microphones into casts of actual pinnae held on a bar without a model of the head in between them. The sounds picked up by the microphones were played to the subjects via high-fidelity headphones. Thus the subjects had remotely controlled but realistic outer ears! The subjects were able to make reasonably accurate judgements of both azimuth (left–front–right, etc.) and elevation. When the pinnae were removed from the microphones, judgements were quite erratic. It is noteworthy that with the artificial pinnae in place subjects reported that the sounds were actually localised out 'in space' and not, as is usually the case with headphones, simply lateralised inside the head. This impression persisted even when one microphone was disconnected. Clearly, then, the pinnae are providing some information as to the location of sound sources. In order to demonstrate more clearly that the pattern of temporal delays was the crucial factor, Batteau constructed a set of time delays artificially using a delay-line. Signals were fed directly to the ear canal via tubes. The signals conveyed an impression of locale which could be altered by adjusting the pattern of delays. Thus the presence of such time-delayed replications seems to be a sufficient condition for the perception of direction.

A number of other experiments have indicated that the pinnae can play a role in sound localisation. Freedman and Fisher (1968) investigated the localisation of short bursts of white noise presented in an acoustically treated room. They compared three conditions: (1) with subjects listening normally, (2) with sound conducted directly to the ears via 10 cm metal tubes and (3) with casts of pinnae on the ends of the tubes. If head movements were restricted there was no significant difference between (1) and (3), while both produced significantly more accurate localisation than did (2). However, if head movements were allowed, there were no differences between the three conditions, all subjects achieving nearly perfect performance. While this experiment demonstrates pinna effects, the accuracy required was not great ($22\frac{1}{2}$ degrees), and the effects were not important when head movements were allowed. It is of interest that in condition (3) the casts were not of the subject's own pinnae. Pinnae differ considerably between people, and it would be of interest to know how far we are able to use, or to learn to use, information from other people's pinnae!

It is clear from these experiments that the encoding action of the pinna can indicate the direction of a sound source. However, the real importance of this coding is still a matter of debate. Most of the experiments investigating monaural localisation have used widely spaced loudspeakers, so that acuities of the order of 1–2 degrees, which can be achieved under binaural conditions, could not have been measured. Further, pinna encoding effects can only be of importance when the stimuli contain high-frequency components; only for frequencies above about 6 kHz is the wavelength of the sound sufficiently short to produce strong interactions with the pinna. However, some pinna effects have been found for frequencies lower than this. Gardner and Gardner (1973) investigated localisation in the median plane for wide-band noise and for bands of noise with various different centre frequencies. They found that occlusion of the pinnae cavities (filling them with moulded rubber plugs) decreased localisation abilities, the largest effects occurring for wide-band noise and for the bands of noise with highest centre frequencies (8 and 10 kHz), although there was still some effect at 3 kHz.

One problem with Batteau's theory of time-delay encoding is that the time delays involved are exceedingly small; 100 to 300 μs is a typical value given by Batteau. While the auditory system is capable of dealing with such time differences for stimuli presented to opposite ears, it is unlikely that the system could resolve two stimuli arriving at the same ear when they are separated by only 100 μs. However, the time delays described by Batteau would not only alter the temporal structure of the stimuli; they would also modify the effective spectrum of the stimuli reaching the ear-drum. Depending on the particular time delays which were present, certain frequency bands would be boosted, while others would be reduced in intensity. This has been confirmed by measurements at the entrance to the ear canal of human observers (Blauert, 1969/1970). The head and pinna together form a filter which is something like a 'comb' filter. Further, the frequency bands which are boosted depend on the direction of sound incidence. Blauert has shown that the perceived direction of the sound source depends upon these boosted bands and that there is relatively little variation between observers in these kinds of judgements. If both ears are stimulated with identical narrow-band noise signals, the direction of the sound sensation depends upon frequency only, and not upon the direction of sound incidence. Similar kinds of results have been found by Butler (1971) for the localisation of tone bursts with one ear occluded. The perceived direction of the sound source depends on frequency, rather than on the actual location of the sound source. While the effects described by Batteau are limited to frequencies above 6 kHz, effects related to the modification of the spectrum of the stimulus may operate at much lower frequencies than this, because the head, as well as the pinnae, can affect the spectrum. The effects described by Blauert and by Butler were found for frequencies between 500 Hz and 16 kHz. We may conclude that while the presence of time-delayed replications is a sufficient condition for the perception of direction, it is not a necessary one. It seems likely that observers are actually processing information relating to the spectrum of the stimulus, and that time delays are only effective by virtue of the spectral changes which they produce.

If the listener is to make efficient use of spectral cues associated with the direction of a sound source, then he must be able to distinguish spectral peaks and dips related to direction from peaks and dips inherent in the character of the stimulus itself. Thus one might expect that a knowledge of the sound source and room conditions may also be important. To some extent, the two ears provide separate sets of spectral cues, so that the difference between the two ears could be used to locate unfamiliar sound sources, but for sound sources in the median plane (i.e. sound sources which are equidistant from the two ears) the cues at the two ears will be identical for all locations. Plenge (1972, 1974) has presented evidence that we do, in fact, make comparisons with stored stimulus patterns in judging the location of a sound source. He showed that if subjects were not allowed to become familiar with the characteristics of the sound source and the listening room, then localisation was disturbed. In many cases the sound sources were lateralised in the head rather than being localised externally. This was particularly true for sound in the median plane. However, such familiarity does not seem to require an extended learning process. We become familiar with sound source characteristics and room acoustics within a very few seconds of entering a new situation.

5.5 THE PRECEDENCE EFFECT

In a normal listening environment the sound from a given source such as a loudspeaker, reaches our ears via a number of different paths. Some of the sound will arrive by a direct path, but a good deal of it will only reach our ears after one or more reflections from the surfaces of the room. In spite of this, we are not normally aware of these reflections, or echoes, and they do not appear to influence our judgements of the direction of the sound source. Thus we are still able accurately to locate a speaker in a reverberant room where the total energy in the reflected sound may be greater than that eaching our ears by a direct path.

Wallach, Newman and Rosenzweig (1949) investigated the way the auditory system copes with echoes in experiments using both sound sources in free space and sounds delivered by headphones. In

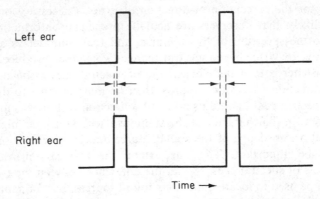

Figure 5.3 The stimulus sequence used by Wallach *et al.* (1949) to investigate the precedence effect. The first pair of clicks arrive at the ears with a small interaural time disparity, indicated by the arrows. The second pair of clicks simulate a room echo and have a different interaural disparity. The whole stimulus sequence is heard as a single sound whose location is determined primarily by the interaural delay of the leading pair of clicks.

the experiments using headphones pairs of clicks were delivered to each ear (two clicks in each earphone). The delay between the two clicks in a pair, and the time of arrival of the first click in a pair could be varied independently (see Figure 5.3). The results can be summarised as follows.

(1) Two brief sounds that reach an observer's ears in close succession will be heard as a single sound if the interval between them is sufficiently short. The interval over which fusion takes place is not the same for all types of sounds. The upper limit of the interval is about 5 ms for single clicks, but may be as long as 40 ms for sounds of a complex character, such as speech or music.

(2) If two brief sounds are heard as fused into a single sound, the location of the total sound is determined largely by the location of the first sound. This is known as the precedence effect.

(3) The effect is only shown for sounds of a discontinuous or transient character.

(4) The second sound, or echo, can be shown to have a small but demonstrable effect. If the location of the second sound departs more and more from the location of the first sound, it will pull the total sound along with it up to a maximal amount (about 7 degrees) and then it becomes progressively less effective.

(5) If the interval between the arrival of the two sounds is 1 ms or less, the precedence effect does not operate; some average or compromise location will be heard.

(6) If the second sound is made sufficiently intense (15 dB above the first sound), it overrides the precedence factor.

(7) The precedence effect is favoured for sounds which are qualitatively similar; if the 'echo' differs greatly from the leading sound, then fusion will not occur.

The precedence effect seems to be essentially a binaural phenomenon; it is the interaural differences in the leading sound which allow an accurate assessment of its location in the presence of echos. The fusion effect itself also seems to depend on binaural interaction. A simple demonstration of this may be obtained by placing one finger in an ear while listening to a speaker in a reverberant room; immediately the characteristics of the room become more apparent. The sound becomes 'muddy' and booming, and it is difficult to locate the speaker accurately. Batteau (1968) has reported that filling the pinnae with silicone rubber produces an increase in subjective amount of reverberation, possibly indicating that pinna encoding effects are also involved. However, no formal experiments on this topic have been reported.

It is clear that the precedence effect plays an important role in our perception of everyday sounds. It enables us to locate, interpret and identify sounds in spite of wide variations in the acoustical conditions in which we hear them. Without it listening in reverberant rooms would be an extremely confusing experience. Sometimes, on the other hand, the effect can be an inconvenience! An example of this is found in the stereophonic reproduction of music. Contrary to popular opinion, the stereo information on a record is coded almost entirely in terms of intensity differences in the two channels; time disparities are eliminated as far as possible, because these would only provide meaningful information for one particular separation of the loudspeakers. If the sound originates in one channel only, then the sound will be clearly located towards that channel. If the sound is equally intense in both channels, then the sound will be located in the centre, between the two channels, provided that the loudspeakers are equidistant from the listener. If, however, the listener is slightly closer to one loudspeaker than to the other, the sound from that loudspeaker will reach him earlier in time, and if the time disparity exceeds 1 ms, the precedence effect will operate; the sound will appear to originate entirely from the nearer loudspeaker. In a normal room this gives the listener a latitude of about 2 ft (60 cm) on either side of the central position. Deviations greater than this will produce significant changes in the 'stereo image'. Almost all of the sound (except that originating entirely from the farther loudspeaker) will appear to come from the closer loudspeaker. Thus the notion of the 'stereo seat' is quite close to the truth. Recently attempts have been made to broaden the acceptable listening area, using 'omnidirectional' loudspeakers, which radiate sound in all directions rather than beaming it forward. It is claimed that with these loudspeakers the listening position is not critical, but many listeners have complained that they are unable to locate a sound source precisely with these loudspeakers no matter where they sit. Clearly, further research is needed before the benefits, if any, of these loudspeakers can be evaluated. This point is discussed further in Section 7.3.

5.6 TIME–INTENSITY TRADING

If identical clicks are presented to the two ears via headphones, then the sound source is usually located in the middle of the head; the image is said to be centred. If now the click in the left ear is made to lead that in the right ear by, say, 100 μs, the sound image will move to the left. However, by making the click in the right ear more intense, it is possible to make the sound image move back towards the right, so that once again the image is centred. Thus it seems possible to trade a time difference at the two ears for an intensity difference.

This finding led to the theory that time differences and intensity differences are eventually coded in the nervous system in a similar sort of way. In particular, it was suggested that the latency of neural responses was shorter to more intense sounds, so that intensity differences were transformed into time differences at the neural level. Thus Deatherage and Hirsh (1957) stated: '. . . once the frame of reference becomes neural, we would hypothesize that intensity, having made its contribution to neural time, may drop out of consideration, leaving the judgement of localization almost entirely dependent upon results of comparison of neural time'.

Many investigators have measured the value of the time–intensity trade, expressed in μs/dB, for different types of stimuli. It is clear that the results are affected by many different variables, including absolute intensity, frequency or frequency band, duration, presence of noise, etc. Thus reported values of the trading function have varied from 1.7 μs/dB for pure tones (Shaxby and Gage, 1932), to 100 μs/dB for pulse trains (Christman and Victor, 1955). Harris (1960) measured the trading relation for clicks which had been high- or low-pass filtered at various cut-off frequencies. He found that low-pass clicks, with cut-off frequencies below 1500 Hz, gave values of about 25 μs/dB, whereas high-pass clicks gave values of about 90 μs/dB. At low sensation levels (20 dB) a discontinuity was apparent at about 1500 Hz, but this disappeared at higher levels. He also noted that when an image is centred by offsetting an intensity difference with a time difference, the variability of the judgements is greater than when sounds equal in intensity are centred. Thus it seems that time differences and intensity differences may not be truly equivalent.

More recently a number of workers have reported that both for tones of low frequency and for clicks observers may report two separate sound images. For tones Whitworth and Jeffress (1961) found that one sound, the 'time image', was little affected by inter-aural differences in level, and showed a trading ratio of about 1 μs/dB. The other, the 'intensity image', showed a trading ratio of about 20 μs/dB. For clicks Hafter and Jeffress (1968) found ratios of 2 to 35 μs/dB for the 'time image,' and 85 to 150 μs/dB for the 'intensity image'. Recently Hafter and Carrier (1972) have confirmed that observers are able to detect differences between diotic signals (identical in each ear) and dichotic signals which have been centred by opposing a time difference with an intensity difference. Thus these experiments confirm that time and intensity differences are not truly equivalent. Notice that in a normal listening situation time and intensity differences would not be opposed. Presumably the perceptual mechanism expects them to covary in a physically realistic fashion, and it is only when this does not occur that two sound images are perceived.

Jeffress (1971) has suggested that there are at least two mechanisms underlying localisation (and lateralisation), one of which is affected by interaural differences in both level and time, operates over the whole of the auditory range and is responsible for the intensity image. The other is little affected by differences in level, but operates on inter-aural time differences over the frequency range below 1500 Hz. This suggestion of a dual mechanism agrees well with the generalisations

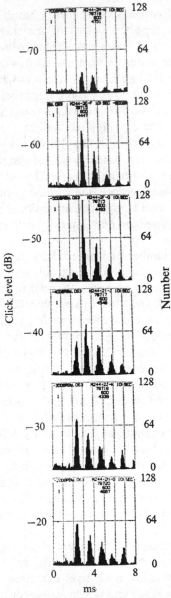

Figure 5.4 Post-stimulus time (PST) histograms of the response to click stimulation of a single auditory nerve fibre, as a function of click level. Each histogram shows the number of nerve firings occurring at a particular time after the instant of click presentation. The CF of the neurone was 630 Hz. Click level is expressed relative to a high reference level, the higher click levels being at the bottom of the figure. From Kiang *et al.* (1965), by permission of the author and M.I.T. Press.

made earlier in this chapter. When we discussed the experiments of Yost *et al.* (1971) on the lateralisation of filtered clicks, we saw that the most accurate localisation was possible when energy was present below 1500 Hz, since in that frequency range the timing of the 'fine-structure' of the waveform on the basilar membrane can be compared at the two ears. For frequencies above this the fine-structure information will be lost, and only the envelopes of the waveforms on the basilar membrane will be compared. Physiological evidence (Kiang *et al.*, 1965) indicates that changes in the intensity of clicks produce relatively little change in latency for those (lower-frequency) fibres which display phase-locking; firings still occur at a particular point on a positive-going deflection of the basilar membrane. However, relatively more responses tend to occur on the first few deflections of the basilar membrane (recall that a click produces a waveform resembling a decaying sinusoidal oscillation), so that the mean latency of neural response, a measure related more to the envelope of the signal, is shorter. This is illustrated in Figure 5.4.

There is, then, some physiological support for Jeffress's suggestion of two central mechanisms. One, the time mechanism, will operate on the time differences in firing of phase-locked neural fibres, which are little affected by changes in level. The second, the intensity mechanism, will be affected both by interaural time differences and by differences in the mean latency of neural response to impulsive signals which result from interaural level differences. We may assume that dual localisations in trading experiments result from conflicts between the two systems.

Taken together, the results of trading experiments make it quite clear that there is not a single simple trade between time and intensity. Rather there appear to be two difference mechanisms by which time and intensity differences interact. However, it is only in the rather artificial situation of the laboratory that these two mechanisms produce sound images in widely different locations. In real life time and intensity differences will nearly always work in conjunction to provide a single, well-defined sound image.

5.7 GENERAL CONCLUSIONS ON SOUND LOCALISATION

We have seen that the human observer is capable of using a great variety of physical cues in determining the location of sound source. Time differences at the two ears, intensity differences at the two ears, changes in the spectral composition of sounds due to head-shadow and pinna effects, and changes in all of these cues produced by head or sound source movements, can all influence the perceived direction of a sound source. In laboratory studies usually just one or two of these cues are isolated. In this way it has been shown that sometimes a single cue may be sufficient for accurate localisation of a sound source. In other experiments one cue has been opposed by another, in order to investigate the relative importance of the cues, or to determine whether the cues are encoded along some common neural dimension. These experiments have shown that, in some senses, the cues are not equivalent, but, on the other hand, they may also not be independent. For real sound sources, such as speech or music, all of the cues described above may be available simultaneously. However, in this situation they will not provide conflicting cues; rather the multiplicity of cues will render the location of the sound sources more sure and more accurate.

5.8 BINAURAL MASKING LEVEL DIFFERENCES

We pointed out earlier that separation of sound sources was one of the benefits of auditory localisation. We will now turn to a group of laboratory experiments which have explored the psychoacoustical basis of such separation in considerable detail. Consider the situation shown in Figure 5.5(a). White noise from the same noise generator is fed to both ears via stereo headphones. Pure tones, also from the same signal generator, are fed separately to each ear and mixed with the noise. Thus the total signals at the two ears are identical. Assume that the level of the tone is adjusted until it is just masked by the noise, i.e. it is at its masked threshold, and let its level at this point be L_0 dB. Provided that the equipment isolates the versions of the noise and of the tone that each ear will receive, we can invert the signal (the tone) in phase at one ear only (this is equivalent to turning the waveform upside-down; see Figure 5.5b). The result is that the tone becomes audible again. The tone can be adjusted to a new level, L_π, so that it is once again at its masked threshold. The difference between the two levels, $L_0 - L_\pi$ (dB) is known as a masking level difference (MLD), and its value may be as large as 15 dB at low frequencies (around 500 Hz), decreasing to 2–3 dB for frequencies above 1500 Hz. Thus simply by inverting the signal waveform at one ear we can make the signal considerably more easy to detect.

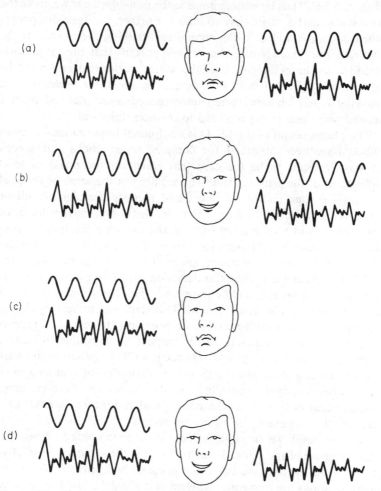

Figure 5.5 Illustration of two situations in which binaural masking-level differences (BMLDs) occur. In conditions (a) and (c) detectability is poor, while in conditions (b) and (d), where the interaural relations of the signal and masker are different, detectability is good (hence the smiling faces).

An example which is perhaps even more startling is given in Figure 5.5(c). The noise and signal are fed to one ear only, and the signal is adjusted to be at its masked threshold. Now the noise alone is added at the other ear; the tone becomes audible once again!

191

(Figure 5.5d). Thus by adding noise at the non-signal ear we make the tone considerably more easy to detect. Further, the tone disappears when it, too, is added to the second ear, making the sounds at the two ears the same. Notice that it is important that the same noise is added to the non-signal ear; the noises at the two ears must be correlated or derived from the same noise generator. Release from masking is not obtained when uncorrelated noise (derived from a second noise generator) is added to the non-signal ear.

The phenomenon of the MLD is not limited to pure tones. Similar effects have been observed for complex tones, clicks and speech sounds. It seems to be the case that whenever the phase or level differences of the signal at the two ears are not the same of those of the masker, our ability to detect and identify the signals will be improved relative to the case where the signal and masker have the same phase and level relationships at the two ears. Such differences will only occur in real situations when the signal and masker are located in different positions in space. Thus one implication of the MLD phenomenon is that the detection and interpretation of signals, including speech, will be improved when the signal and masker are not coincident in space. The MLD is thus seen to be very closely related to the 'cocktail-party' phenomenon. However, it appears that the MLD is not merely another aspect of our ability to localise sounds, because the largest MLDs occur with the situation of phase inversion (see above) which only occurs naturally for mid-frequency pure tones at highly restricted angular locations. Further, large MLDs occur in situations where the signal and masker are not subjectively well separated in space (see below).

At this point we must introduce some terminology. When the relative phase of the signal at the two ears is the same as the relative phase of the masker, the condition is called homophasic. When the phase relations are opposite, the term 'antiphasic' is used. In general we can describe a particular situation by using the symbols N (for noise) and S (for signal), each being followed by a suffix denoting relative phase at the two ears. A phase reversal is equivalent to a phase shift of 180 degrees or π radians. Thus $N_0 S_\pi$ refers to the condition where the noise is in phase at the earphones and the signal is reversed in phase. In general, this leads to the largest MLDs, although $N_\pi S_0$ is also large.

A number of models have been presented which attempt to account for the MLD phenomenon. In general, these have not attempted explanations at the physiological level, but have rather been 'black-box' models, assuming that the auditory system is capable of certain types of processing without specifying exactly how it is done. Before we discuss these models we shall present some of the experimental findings which the models have to explain.

5.8.1 *The MLD as an empirical phenomenon*

One very general finding which has emerged from MLD studies is that the largest effects occur at low frequencies. Effects greater than 2–3 dB are limited to the frequency region below about 1500 Hz, and it is noteworthy that this is also the highest frequency for which we are able to compare phases at the two ears in localising sounds. Thus it is likely that the MLD depends at least in part on the transmission of temporal information about the stimulus to some higher neural centre which compares the temporal information from the two ears.

A second general feature which has emerged is that for a wide-band masker not all of the frequency components are effective; just as was the case for normal masking (see Chapter 3), only those components in a critical band around the signal seem to be effective in masking it. Mulligan, Mulligan and Stonecypher (1967) presented a tone to one ear only and investigated the effects of various different masking noises at the two ears. They found that so long as the critical band levels at the two ears remained the same, changes in the masker's bandwidth and overall level at one ear, with respect to the other, had no effect on detection. In other words, only changes within the critical band affected the detectability of the tone. A narrow band of noise at the non-signal ear was sufficient to provide release from masking produced by a wider band of correlated noise (derived from the same noise generator) at the other ear, but no release was observed when the noise was uncorrelated.

In addition to improving the detectability of tones, conditions which produce MLDs also favour other aspects of our ability to analyse signals. For example, when speech signals are presented against noisy backgrounds, we may be able to detect that something was said, but not to identify what was said. In such situations a number of workers have shown improved speech intelligibility under antiphasic conditions (e.g. Hirsh, 1950). More recently Gebhardt and Goldstein (1972) measured frequency DLs for tones presented against noise backgrounds and found that, for a given signal-to-noise ratio, antiphasic DLs are substantially smaller than homophasic ones when the signals are close to masked threshold. Thus antiphasic conditions improve our ability to identify and discriminate signals, as well as to detect them.

The relative importance of spatial factors in the MLD was investigated by Carhart, Tillman and Greetis (1969). They measured thresholds for spondees and monosyllables in the presence of four competing maskers, a situation which mirrors the 'cocktail-party' phenomenon quite closely. Two of the maskers were modulated white noise and two were whole sentences. They used several different listening conditions, including homophasic, antiphasic and those where the signal or the maskers were delayed at one ear relative to the other. In these latter conditions the different maskers were sometimes given opposing time delays, so that some would be located towards one ear and some towards the other. Sometimes the signal was subjectively well-separated in location from the masking sounds, and under these conditions subjects reported the task of identifying the spondees to be easier. However, the largest MLDs were obtained for the antiphasic condition, where there is no clear separation in the subjective locations; rather the sound images are located diffusely within the head. Thus escape from masking and lateralisation/localisation seem, to some extent, to be separate capacities.

Recently it has been reported that MLDs occur for both forward and backward masking (Small *et al.*, 1972; Dolan and Trahiotis, 1972). Substantial MLDs (4–5 dB) are found for silent intervals between the signal and the masker of up to 40 ms. Thus it seems that detailed aspects of the waveforms at the two ears (such as phase) are retained in the auditory system until interaction between the signal and masker occurs.

5.9 MODELS TO EXPLAIN MLDs

Although a large number of models have been proposed to account for the MLD, none is completely successful in explaining all aspects of the experimental data. We shall discuss the two models which have been the most influential in this area, and follow this with a more general discussion.

5.9.1 *The Webster–Jeffress model*

Webster (1951) pointed out that a narrow-band noise resembles a sinusoid whose amplitude and phase vary slowly from moment to moment. The band of noise which is effective in masking the tone, the critical band, may also be thought of in this way. Adding a tonal signal to this noise will yield a resultant which generally will differ in phase and amplitude from the original noise. If, for example, adding the signal at one ear advances the signal plus noise in phase, adding the signal reversed in phase at the other ear will retard it. This is illustrated in Figure 5.6(a). The effects may be illustrated graphically at one instant in time by a vector diagram (Figure 5.6b). The noise is represented by a vector whose length denotes the amplitude and whose angle denotes a phase. The signal is denoted by a second vector, whose length again denotes amplitude, but which generally differs in phase from the noise by an angle α. The figure shows the case where an antiphasic signal is added to a narrow band of noise in phase at the two ears. It may be seen that the resultant leads in phase at one ear and also has a greater amplitude at that ear. With a noise-masker and a tonal signal the phase angle of addition, α, will vary constantly, so that the differences in level and phase at the two ears will vary from moment to moment. In some cases one ear will lead in time but the other will receive the more intense stimulus.

According to the Webster–Jeffress model, binaural detection is based upon the differences in phase and level at the two ears which result from the addition of the signal to the band of frequencies in the noise which contribute to the masking of the signal. Thus the cues for detection will be similar to those involved in the ordinary localisation and lateralisation of binaural signals.

Jeffress and his colleagues (e.g. McFadden, Jeffress and Ermey, 1972) have described a series of experiments on MLDs where the phase angle between the signal and noise, α, was controlled, thus controlling the relative magnitude of the interaural time and level differences. They used a rather special stimulus situation, where both signal and masker were the same narrow band of noise. When α is 0 degrees, the signal is added to the masker in one ear and subtracted in the other. There is no interaural phase difference, but the level difference is maximal. For this condition substantial MLDs (up to 15 dB) occurred for frequencies of 250, 1000 and 2000 Hz. When α is 90 degrees, the signal vectors are at right angles to the

13-2

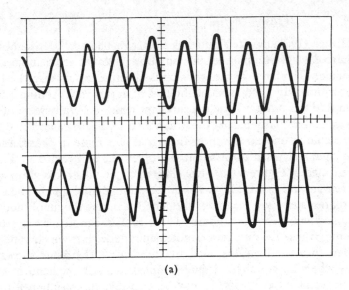

(a)

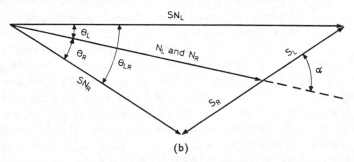

(b)

Figure 5.6 In (a) oscilloscope traces of the signals presented to the left ear (upper) and right ear (lower) are shown. For the first part of the trace only a narrow-band noise, identical in the two channels, is present. Then a tonal signal, reversed in phase in one channel relative to the other, is added. Note the resultant phase and amplitude shift between the two channels. In (b) the situation at one instant in time is represented by a vector diagram. The in-phase narrow-band noise is represented by N_L and N_R. The signal in the left ear is denoted by S_L, and the signal in the right ear, which is opposite in phase, by S_R. The phase angle of addition, α, would vary randomly from moment to moment. Note that the resultant in the left ear, SN_L, differs from the resultant in the right ear, SN_R, in both amplitude and phase. From Jeffress (1971), by permission of the author.

masker vector, so that the interaural phase difference is a maximum, but there is no interaural level difference. For this condition large MLDs were found for frequencies of 250, 500 and 1000 Hz, but not for 2000 Hz. For α between 90 and 180 degrees the ear that is leading in time will receive the weaker stimulus. Thus time and intensity will be in opposition. Substantial MLDs were still found, although the subjects were sometimes not able to lateralise the signal clearly to one side. This inability to lateralise is probably not due to a cancellation of time and intensity; as we discussed earlier, the subjects will tend to hear two sound images, so that responses are inconsistent.

Jeffress (1971) has summarised these results as follows: 'Detection thus appears to be an aspect of lateralization. The signal is detected because it is heard as a displacement from the noise in the median plane. Even when time and level are in opposition there is movement away from the median plane, a movement which is detectable although ambiguous in direction.' Subjects differ in their sensitivity to the two cues, time and level differences, and at 2000 Hz only level differences can be used.

Clearly, this model, when applied to the particular stimuli used by Jeffress, does explain the data rather well. However, the use of the same stimulus as both a signal and masker is a rather special case. For a tonal signal presented against a wide-band random noise, the phase angle α will vary randomly from moment to moment. Thus the subjective lateral position of the signal-plus-noise (the noise here referring to those components in a critical band around the tone) will also vary randomly from moment to moment. This does not fit in with observers' reports. Rather, if the tone can be faintly heard, it will be lateralised fairly precisely in one position. Thus for the $N_0 S_\pi$ condition, the noise will generally be lateralised in the middle of the head, whereas the tone will be heard towards one side. For their narrow-band signals and maskers McFadden, Jeffress and Ermey (1971) state that 'the phenomenology associated with detecting an S_π signal is that during a signal-plus-masker trial, there is a slight movement or shift in the auditory "image" '. If the model applied equally well to a tonal signal in wide-band noise, then a part of the sound image should be heard as fluctuating in position. This does not seem to be the case.

The model also cannot explain the finding of MLDs in forward and backward masking. In order for the vector addition of signal and masker to occur, these must be present simultaneously. Thus the model deals rather well with some specific stimulus situations, but fails to account for the data in others.

5.9.2 *Durlach's equalisation and cancellation model*

This mathematical model, presented by Durlach (1963), has four basic components, which are illustrated in Figure 5.7. First, the stimulus in each ear is assumed to be filtered, by a mechanism analogous to the critical band. Then the total output from one filter is transformed relative to that at the other filter in such a way that the masking components become the same in both channels (the E process). The signal in one channel is then subtracted from that in the other (the C process), thus eliminating the masking signal. If the interaural relations of the signal are different from those of the masker, then some of the signal will remain after the C process, so that if precision is perfect, the signal-to-noise ratio is improved by an infinite amount. The output from the EC mechanism is fed to a decision device which also receives inputs directly from the band-pass filters. It is assumed that the subject's detection performance is determined by the largest signal-to-noise ratio at the inputs to the decision device. The ratio at the binaural input (from the EC mechanism), divided by the ratio at one of the monaural inputs, is called the 'EC factor', and describes the change in masked threshold produced by the binaural processing.

Clearly, human observers do not show infinite MLDs. In order to account for this, it is assumed that the EC process is performed imperfectly, so that there will be a residue of noise at the output of the C mechanism. The imperfections are assumed to be of two types: (1) those resulting from a random jitter independent of stimulus configuration, and representable as random errors in the amplitude and time alignment of the signals at the input to the C mechanism; (2) those resulting from 'atypical' stimuli that require atypical E transformations in response. Examples of the second type might be broadband masking signals that differ by an interaural phase shift rather than an interaural time shift, or signals that differ by an interaural time shift greater than the time it takes a sound to travel around the head.

It is assumed that there are a number of possible modes of operation of the EC mechanism, but that a selector mechanism chooses

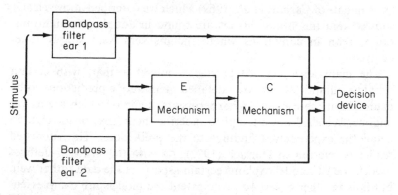

Figure 5.7 Illustration of the major components in Durlach's (1963) equalisation and cancellation model of binaural processing.

that mode which gives the best 'EC factor'. It is usually assumed that the types of operation which the E mechanism can perform are those which would be involved in the localisation or lateralisation of sounds, namely shifts in time and shifts in intensity. For a tone a phase shift is equivalent to a time shift, and for a narrow-band noise this is also approximately true. Thus for the $N_\pi S_0$ condition the appropriate E process will be a shift in time of the noise components around the tone. Since a narrow-band noise resembles a sinusoid, a shift in time equal to half a period of the sinusoid will be equivalent to inverting the phase.

A problem arises when we consider antiphasic conditions for wide-band signals, such as speech sounds, in wide-band maskers. If, for example, the noise is inverted in one ear with respect to the other, a shift in time will only cancel the noise components in certain frequency regions, while in other frequency regions the noise will actually be increased. Further, such a shift in time will tend to cancel the signal components in certain frequency regions. Since substantial MLDs do occur under these conditions, we must assume either that different time shifts are used in different frequency bands, or that the E mechanism is capable of a rather strange and demanding operation —that of inverting a waveform. It would seem reasonable that if such complicated transformations are required of the E mechanism, then the MLDs would be *smaller* than those found in the case where, for example, the masker in one ear is simply delayed in time with respect to the other. However, this does not seem to be the case. The experiments of Carhart *et al.* (1969) which we described above clearly showed that the largest MLDs are found in antiphasic conditions, rather than in conditions where the maskers were simply time-delayed.

The main advantage of Durlach's model is that, with certain simple assumptions, it allows detailed quantitative predictions to be made about the outcome of experiments, some of which are as yet undone. We shall not attempt to describe these here, or to relate in detail the experimental findings to the predictions. The interested reader is referred to Durlach (1972). As with the Webster–Jeffress model, the EC model explains certain aspects of the data rather well, but fails in other cases. To some extent the models are complementary, each one being able to explain some of the results which do not fit the other. The EC model provides the best fit to data on the detection of signals in wide-band maskers, whereas the Webster–Jeffress model provides the better explanation for narrow-band signals and maskers. Neither model can satisfactorily explain the finding of MLDs in forward and backward masking, although the EC model could be extended to do this.

5.10 GENERAL DISCUSSION

Although the models we have described are by no means the only explanations of MLDs that have been published, they are fairly typical of work in this area. The main difference in the models is in their emphasis; the Webster–Jeffress model is more concerned with explanations in terms of the characteristics of the signals themselves, whereas the EC model is more concerned with the types of operation that the observer might be able to perform in detecting binaural signals. Neither model is completely satisfactory in providing a description of the subjective experiences that accompany binaural detection. As Durlach (1972) has said of the EC model, 'although the primary purpose of the model is to describe objective performance and not the subjective experience, it would obviously be more satisfactory if the model seemed less artificial when compared with this experience'.

A second limitation of the models is that they were designed only to account for detection performance, and not for the improvements that occur in the discrimination of above-threshold signals. Durlach (1972) has pointed out that the EC model can be extended to account for binaural phenomena other than improved detection, but as yet neither the EC model nor the Webster–Jeffress model can account for the improved intelligibility of speech sounds which occurs under antiphasic conditions.

It is likely that factors other than the MLD play a role in listening situations involving competing sources of stimulation. One of these we have already mentioned: the experiment of Broadbent and Ladefoged (1957) showing that for harmonic complex tones perceptual fusion or separation depends on whether the harmonics are multiples of a single fundamental frequency or of two different fundamental frequencies. In terms of the 'cocktail-party' problem, this means that provided two voices do not have the same fundamental frequency, or larynx tone, these voices will be heard as separate perceptual entities, and there will be little confusion between them.

The results we have been discussing have certain implications for the design and fitting of hearing aids. Firstly, head movements play a significant role in our ability to localise sounds and to understand speech in noisy environments (Hirsh, 1971). For this to benefit the hearing-aid wearer, the aid must be mounted on the head, not the body. Secondly, binaural cues improve sound localisation and allow the MLD effect to operate. Thus, for a person deaf in both ears, two head-worn hearing-aids are needed. Two hearing-aids will also avoid the loss of signal due to head shadow effects. Thirdly, the use of two hearing-aids will enable the precedence effect to operate, so that the listener will be less susceptible to room echos. Fourthly, if the pick-up is actually mounted in the middle ear, advantage can be taken of the encoding effects of the pinna. The extent to which these factors are important will vary with different types of deafness, and will also depend on the quality of the hearing-aid. Attempts to demonstrate the 'cocktail-party' effect using conventional hearing-aids have proved difficult (Kuyper and de Boer, 1969), although significant improvements in intelligibility do result if signals are fed to the hearing-aids via high-quality microphones (Kuyper, 1972). It is likely that the advantages to be gained from MLD effects will not be fully realised with conventional hearing-aids unless their low-frequency response is considerably improved. Similar limitations would presumably apply to the use of pinna encoding effects, except that here an extended high-frequency response would be required, which is often not utilisable by the subject requiring an aid.

For many patients head-worn aids are not practicable, because the high level of amplification required can only be provided by a body-worn aid. However, for such patients significant advantages can be gained by using two separate hearing-aids, one feeding each ear. Byrne and Dermody (1975) showed that localisation of sound with binaural body-worn hearing-aids was far superior to localisation with monaural body-worn aids. Heyes and Ferris (1975) presented similar results, although they found that post-aural aids produced better localisation than body-worn aids, and that a single post-aural aid was about as good as a pair of chest-mounted aids. They concluded that 'a single chest-mounted aid is so poor that for those hearing-aid users for whom sound localisation is important, for example, the blind, its provision should be regarded as a last resort'.

5.11 THE INFLUENCE OF VISION ON AUDITORY LOCALISATION

Many everyday experiences indicate that auditory localisation can be influenced by conflicting visual cues. At a cinema the loudspeakers are usually placed behind the screen, in its centre (except where stereo or multichannel sound is used), yet the sound still appears to come from the actor's mouth as he moves about the screen. Similarly, the loudspeaker in a television set is usually located to one side of the screen, but the sound does not appear to be 'detached' from the visual image.

A number of experiments in recent years have shown that exposure to conflicting auditory and visual cues for a period of time may lead to an after-effect in which the localisation of sounds is systematically displaced. This does not indicate that the whole of our capacity for auditory localisation is learned; indeed the ability to locate sounds seems to be present very early in life, so that a sharp click may elicit an appropriate orienting response from a baby a few minutes after birth (Peiper, 1963). However, it may be the case that connections between the 'frames of reference' for auditory space and for spaces in other modalities (visual, vestibular and kinesthetic) may be modifiable to some extent.

Young (1928) and later Willey, Inglis and Pearce (1937) attempted to distort auditory space using a pseudophone, by which a tube from each ear is led to a trumpet on the opposite side of the head. With this arrangement, sounds from the left are heard as coming from the right, and vice versa. Although the listeners were able to learn to respond appropriately, no genuine auditory reorientation appeared to take place, even after a week of exposure. Held (1955) used an electronic pseudophone which displaced the interaural axis by 22 degrees about the vertical axis of the head. After wearing this for a day, listeners were tested with the pseudophone set to give no displacement. They reported that a single sound source produced two images, one near the normal position and one displaced from it in the opposite direction to the original direction of rotation of the pseudophone. More recently Kalil and Freedman (1967) found that after wearing a pseudophone which displaced a sound 15 degrees to the right of a visible source, subjects heard a sound presented straight in front of them (from a concealed source) as displaced a few degrees to the left. Freedman, Wilson and Rekosh (1967) have reported similar effects for subjects exposed to discordant auditory and kines thetic cues.

Weerts and Thurlow (1971) suggested that the after-effects might arise from asymmetrical auditory stimulation. However, they found that subjects who are exposed to a sound coming from straight ahead, but who turn their eyes 20 degrees to the side towards a visible loudspeaker, show a shift in the localisation of the sound during presentation, and also a corresponding after-effect. Thus substantial effects can be produced under conditions of symmetrical auditory stimulation. Among subjects who turned their heads to the side, the largest effects were found for those who expected to hear the sound coming from the visible source. Subjects who did not turn their eyes, but were led to expect that the sound would appear to come from a loudspeaker 20 degrees to one side, showed no significant shift. Thus the results cannot be simply explained in terms of 'suggestion'. Weerts and Thurlow carried out a number of further experiments in an attempt to isolate the cause of the shifts in localisation. They found that part, but not all, of the shift during the exposure period can be understood in terms of a shift in perceived head direction. When subjects were asked to indicate their head direction with a flashlight pointer, they showed a slight shift, whether their eyes were open or closed. The after-effects were shown not to be due to a change in physical or perceived eye or head position, or to a shift in felt arm position (when using a pointer). Further, the effects are not due to some distortion of the visual fields, since essentially the same results were obtained for subjects blindfolded during the test conditions.

Thus the most likely explanation of these results does seem to be a sort of 'recalibration' of auditory space on the basis of visual information.

Some experiments of Wallach (1940) also indicate the importance of visual orientation in auditory localisation. His subjects had their heads fixed in the vertical axis of a cylindrical screen which rotated about them. The screen was covered in vertical stripes, and after watching the movement of these for a few moments, the observer would perceive himself as in constant rotation and the screen as at rest. A stationary sound source was then activated straight ahead of the observer. Since the observer in this situation perceives himself as moving, he has to interpret the sound source as lying directly above or below him. If the sound source is at a constant azimuth (e.g. 20 degrees to the left of the observer), the sound source cannot be interpreted as lying above the observer, since interaural differences of time and intensity now exist. Instead the source is perceived as rotating with the listener at an elevation which is approximately the complement of the constant azimuth (in this case at an elevation of about 70 degrees). Thus our interpretation of auditory spatial cues is strongly influenced by our perceived visual orientation. Or, more correctly, the highest level of spatial representation is not unimodal, although visual inputs have the most power to influence it.

5.12 THE PERCEPTION OF DISTANCE

Just as was the case for judgements of lateral position, there are a number of cues which we can use in judging the distance of a sound source. For familiar sounds intensity may give a crude indication of distance from the listener. Over moderate distances the spectrum of a complex sound source may also be changed, owing to the absorbing properties of the air; high frequencies are attenuated more than low. However, judgements will again depend on familiarity with the specific situation (Coleman, 1962, 1963). In addition to these cues, the curvature of the wavefront can indicate the distance of a sound source. When this is nearby, the wavefront will be strongly curved, whereas a distant source will produce a plane wavefront. The curvature can be detected in two ways. One of these is to do with the phase of the particle velocity (of air molecules) with respect to sound pressure. von Békésy (1960) demonstrated the effectiveness of this cue for sounds close to the head, and showed that electronic manipulation of these factors could change the apparent distance of a spark discharge from adjacent to a monaural headphone to as much as 60 cm away. The curvature of the wavefront also influences interaural differences in intensity and time, so that a combination of the information from these two could provide a cue as to distance. The fact that time and intensity fail to trade completely (see Section 5.6) indicates that the time and intensity information is preserved separately in the nervous system, so that in principle judgements of distance could be made. Further, in real life many different time–intensity combinations will occur, depending on the distance of the sound source, but we never perceive two sound 'images'. Thus everyday experience indicates that we combine the information from time and intensity differences to produce a single sound image at a well-defined distance. As yet, however, it has not been clearly demonstrated, in a laboratory situation, that we are able to use interaural time and intensity combinations in judging distance.

So far we have discussed the cues which could be used to judge the distance of a sound source in free space. Normally we listen in rooms with reflecting walls, so that the ratio of direct to reflected sound, and the time delay between direct and reflected sound, provide cues as to distance. von Békésy (1960) showed that altering these ratios produced the impression of sounds moving towards or away from the listener. The work of Wallach *et al.* (1949) on the precedence effect (see above) showed that we exhibit little direct awareness of room echoes; rather these are fused with the leading sound. It seems that we are still able to use information related to echoes, in spite of this perceptual fusion.

We may conclude that, just as was the case for judgements of the direction of sound sources, judgements of distance may depend on a multiplicity of cues. Intensity, spectral changes, curvature of the wavefront and reflected sounds may all influence judgements of distance, and some of these may be strongly affected by familiarity with the sound source and the listening environment. In general, localisation of sounds in depth is relatively inaccurate, and errors of the order of 20 per cent are not uncommon for unfamiliar sound sources.

5.13 OBSTACLE DETECTION AND THE BLIND

It is well known that many blind people, and some sighted people, are able to detect the presence of obstacles in the environment and to judge their distance. However, such people are not often able to explain how they do this, and the descriptions which are used, such as 'feeling the objects on my face', are not particularly helpful. Supa, Cotzin and Dallenbach (1944) carried out a series of experiments to determine the cues involved in what they called 'facial vision'. In an initial experiment they found that blindfolded normal subjects could learn to avoid objects after a short learning period, but that blind subjects could normally detect objects at greater distances. Both normal and blind subjects could distinguish between the first perception of an object at a distance and the 'near approach' to it.

There have been two types of cures suggested as the basis for facial vision. These are cutaneous sensation due to air currents, etc., and auditory sensation based on the reflection of sound from obstacles. Supa *et al.* attempted to eliminate each of these cues in turn; cutaneous cues were removed by covering the skin with veils, sleeves, etc., and auditory cues were removed by plugging the ears or by using a background masking noise. They concluded that stimulation of the face and other areas of the skin is neither a necessary nor a sufficient condition for obstacle detection, whereas aural stimulation is both necessary and sufficient.

These experiments were extended by Cotzin and Dallenbach (1950). They used a sound source, whose movement could be controlled by a listener, with a microphone suspended above it at about ear height. The sound picked up by the microphone was fed to the listener via an earphone, and he was required to report when an obstacle was detected. Both wide-band noise and pure tones were used as stimuli. The authors concluded that: (1) changes in pitch (or in a pitch-like quality for the noise) are a sufficient condition for the detection of an obstacle; (2) changes in loudness are neither necessary nor sufficient; (3) high frequencies (around 10 kHz) are necessary for obstacle detection; and (4) the bases of obstacle detection are pitch changes resulting from a Doppler shift (a change in apparent frequency when the observer and the sound source are in relative motion; an example is the change in pitch of a train whistle as the train approaches and passes a stationary observer).

The pitch changes which Cotzin and Dallenbach suggested as a basis for obstacle detection will only occur when the observer is moving. However, other auditory cues may be available to signal the presence and distance of an obstacle. Wilson (1967) has pointed out that, in the neighbourhood of an obstacle, sound reaches the observer both directly and by reflection from the obstacle. Interference between these signals introduces a series of maxima and minima in the spectrum, the frequencies of which depend on the path difference. For a sound containing a wide range of frequencies a pitch is heard (sometimes called the 'reflection tone') which becomes higher as the obstacle is approached. Thus the value of this pitch, and its rate of change as the obstacle is approached, will provide cues as to the distance of the object. In addition, the spectrum of the reflected sound will be modified according to the size of the obstacle; a large object will reflect both high and low frequencies, whereas a small object will only reflect high frequencies. Thus spectral changes in the reflected sound will provide at least a crude estimate of the size of the object. Further changes in spectrum may result if the obstacle absorbs certain portions of the spectrum, or if it introduces frequency-dependent phase shifts. Thus a crude form of obstacle recognition may even be possible. Tests using blind subjects have shown that objects subtending an angle as small as $3\frac{1}{2}$ degrees can be detected, and that changes in distance of the order of 20 per cent and in area of the order of 30 per cent can be discriminated (Kellog, 1962). Kellog also investigated the discrimination of discs covered with different types of material. He found that some materials could be discriminated with high accuracy (plain wood and velvet could be discriminated 99.5 per cent of the time, while others, such as painted wood and glass, could not be discriminated at all. In general, discrimination was good between 'soft' and 'hard' materials, but, surprisingly, denim cloth and velvet could be distinguished with 86.5 per cent accuracy. Rice (1967) found that some subjects could distinguish between a circle, a square and a triangle of the same surface area with an accuracy of about 80 per cent. In order to achieve these discriminations most subjects emitted both normal vocal sounds and clicking and hissing sounds.

In an attempt to make the auditory correlates of objects and their spatial relationships simpler, and to provide more detailed information, a number of aids for the blind have been developed. One of these consists of a 'torch' which projects a beam of noise into the environment and which can be pointed by the observer so as to scan different objects in the environment. A development of this (Kay, 1966) projects a beam of ultrasonic vibrations, whose reflections are picked up by a receiver on the 'torch' and recoded to provide an audible output through an earpiece. The device is designed so that bleeps are heard whose pitch is directly related to distance from the objects producing the reflections. Because of its very high frequency, the ultrasonic beam behaves almost like a beam of light, so that the device can be used to pick out the silhouette of an object. A possible problem, however, is that the sensory display provided is not consistent with the displays resulting from normal auditory space perception, and facility in use may require long learning. No doubt, further studies of the cues used in obstacle detection will suggest the development of other aids for the blind.

5.14 GENERAL CONCLUSIONS

In this chapter we have discussed the cues and the mechanism involved in the localisation of sounds. Our acuity in locating sounds is greatest in the horizontal dimension, fairly good in the vertical direction and least good in the depth (distance) dimension. For each of these dimensions we are able to use a number of distinct cues, although the cues may differ depending on the type of sound and on the mode of presentation. The multiplicity of cues provides a certain redundancy in the system, so that even under very difficult conditions (reverberant rooms or brief sounds) we are still capable of quite accurate localisation.

Binaural processing, using information relating to the differences of the signals at the two ears, contributes to our ability to localise sounds, and may also improve our ability to detect and analyse signals in noisy backgrounds. This is illustrated by laboratory studies of the binaural masking level difference (MLD), and by the 'cocktail-party' phenomenon. Binaural processing also helps us to suppress room echoes, and to locate sound sources in reverberant rooms.

Our judgements of auditory location may be influenced by visual or kinesthetic stimulation. Such stimulation may also lead to after-effects in which the apparent position of a sound source is slightly displaced from its 'true' position. These effects may indicate that there is some 'plasticity' in the relations between auditory, visual and kinesthetic space, so that a 'recalibration' of auditory space can occur on the basis of information from other modalities.

Blind people, and blindfolded normal subjects after some practice, are able to detect obstacles in the environment, and to make crude estimations of their distance and of their size and nature. This ability depends upon the reflections of sound from the obstacles, although subjects are not always aware of this. Again, a number of possible cues may be used in this situation, but the most important one is probably the 'reflection tone' which results from the interference of direct and reflected sound, and whose pitch depends on path difference.

6

Speech Perception

6.1 INTRODUCTION

In this chapter we shall be concerned with the problem of how the complex acoustical patterns of which speech is composed are transformed at the perceptual level into linguistic units. The details of this process are still not fully understood, in spite of an increasing volume of research over the past thirty years or so. What has become clear is that speech perception does not proceed via simple transformations from physical cues directly available in the acoustic waveform. This has been illustrated both by perceptual studies and by attempts to build machines which recognise speech (see Hyde, 1972). A given speech sound is not represented by a given, fixed acoustic pattern in the speech wave; instead the pattern representing it will vary according to the preceding and following sounds, in a complex manner. This has led to a particular kind of theoretical orientation, according to which speech perception is an active process which involves reference to articulatory mechanisms. This idea has had a widespread influence. A similar theory was described in Chapter 4 in relation to the perception of 'residue' tones. For such tones, which are composed of a number of harmonics of a complex tone, the pitch corresponds to the (missing) fundamental. Thurlow (1963) suggested that this pitch was mediated by vocal activity; the subject produces a matching signal whose fundamental frequency is adjusted so that its harmonics coincide with those of the externally presented tone. The perceived pitch will correspond to that fundamental frequency. According to Thurlow, the vocal activity could be overt or subliminal, or involve only auditory imagery.

Certain theories of speech perception have been advanced which, in their basic assumptions, are similar to Thurlow's theory. Firstly, they emphasise that speech perception is a process involving active matching. Secondly, they emphasise that reference to articulation is involved, although the reference may take place entirely in the nervous system, in terms of the neural commands corresponding to articulation, and may not involve actual muscular movements. And, finally, they state that the perception will correspond to the internally generated matching stimulus rather than to the stimulus which was actually presented. One of the aims of this chapter will be to present the reader with some of the reasons why such theories have been felt to be necessary and to discuss why they have had such an important place in the development of theories of speech perception; Thurlow's mediation hypothesis has had relatively little influence on theories of pitch perception, whereas 'active' theories of speech perception have generated a tremendous amount of discussion and experimental work. A second aim of the chapter will be to assess the extent to which such theories are supported by recent experimental evidence.

It is clear that for connected discourse speech perception does not depend solely on cues present in the acoustic waveform. The linguistic context is also of considerable importance. A word or part of a word which is highly probably in the context of a sentence will be 'heard' when the acoustic cues for that word are minimal or even completely absent. For example, Warren (1970b) has shown that when an extraneous sound (such as a cough) completely replaces a speech sound in a recorded sentence, listeners believe they hear the missing sound. This phenomenon is probably related to the 'pulsation threshold' phenomenon described in Chapter 3; when a weak tone is alternated with a louder tone of similar frequency, the weak tone sounds continuous even though it is, in fact, pulsating. The effect reported by Warren has been shown to depend on similar factors; the listeners only 'hear' the missing sound if the cough is relatively intense and contains frequency components close to those of the missing sound. This kind of filling-in process is obviously of importance when we are listening in noisy environments, and it illustrates the importance of non-acoustic cues in speech perception. On the other hand, we are able to recognise words spoken in isolation, provided they are clearly articulated, so that linguistic context is not a *necessary* requirement for the perception of speech.

It is far beyond the scope of this book to give more than a brief description of certain selected aspects of speech perception. We shall

14-2

ignore entirely the aspects of speech recognition related to semantic cues (the meaning of preceding and following words), syntactic cues (grammatical rules) and circumstantial cues (speaker identity, subject matter, etc.), although these may be of considerable importance, especially in noisy environments. We shall concentrate rather on the processing of cues in the acoustic waveform. The study of these cues has been greatly aided by the use of speech synthesisers. These devices allow the production of acoustic waveforms resembling real speech to a greater or lesser extent; the closeness of the resemblance depends upon the complexity of the device and the trouble to which the experimenter is prepared to go. However, in contrast to real speech, these waveforms have controlled and precisely reproducible characteristics. Using a speech synthesiser, the experimenter can manipulate certain features of the speech wave form, leaving all the other characteristics unchanged, and so he can investigate what aspects of the waveform determine how it will be perceived. The results of such experiments have been instrumental in the formulation of theories of speech perception.

6.2 THE NATURE OF SPEECH SOUNDS

The most familiar units of speech are words, which can often be broken down into somewhat smaller units—that is, into syllables. However, linguists generally consider that even syllables can be analysed in terms of sequences of smaller units—the speech sounds or phonemes. To clarify the nature of phonemes, consider the following examples. The word 'bit' is composed of three phonemes, an initial, a middle and a final element. We use each of these phonemes when we discriminate 'bit' from 'pit', 'bet' and 'bid'. Thus, for the linguist, the phonemes are the basic units of sound that in any given language differentiate one word from another. On their own they do not symbolise any concept or object (many are not even pronounceable in isolation), but in relation to other phonemes they distinguish one word from another, and in combination they form syllables and words. Not all linguists or psychologists would accept that it is appropriate to consider phonemes as 'the basic units' of speech, and indeed a few would deny that the phoneme has any perceptual reality as a unit (e.g. Warren, 1975), since (as we shall see later) some phonemes cannot be heard in isolation. However, the analysis of speech in terms of phonemes has been widespread and influential, and we shall, for the purposes of discussion, continue to use the concept. When a letter is used to represent a phoneme this is indicated by a slash (/) before and after the letter.

The simplest view of speech perception would hold that speech is composed of a series of sounds or acoustic features, and that each feature, or set of features, corresponds to a particular phoneme. Thus the speech sounds would have a one-to-one correspondence with the phonemes, and a sequence of speech sounds would be perceived as a sequence of phonemes, which would then be combined into words and phrases. This view has been seriously challenged, largely as a result of experiments using synthetic speech conducted at the Haskins Laboratories, in the USA. To understand this challenge we must consider in more detail the characteristics of speech sounds.

Figure 6.1 illustrates how the phonemes of English can be classified according to the way in which they are produced by the articulatory apparatus. The section which follows outlines the relationship between the manner of production and the acoustic characteristics of the speech. Speech sounds are produced by the vocal organs, namely the lungs, the windpipe, the larynx (containing the vocal cords), the throat or pharynx, the nose and nasal cavities, and the mouth. The part of this system lying above the larynx is called the vocal tract, and its shape can be varied extensively by movements of various parts such as the tongue, the lips and the jaw. The glottis is an opening at the upper part of the windpipe, between the vocal cords, and it can affect the flow of air from the lungs by opening or closing. The term 'glottal source' refers to the sound energy produced by the flow of air past the vocal cords as they open and close quite rapidly in a periodic or quasi-periodic manner. This produces a periodic complex tone with a relatively low pitch, whose spectrum initially contains energy at harmonics covering a wide range of frequencies. This spectrum is subsequently modified according to the shape of the vocal tract. Speech sounds produced while the vocal cords are vibrating are said to be voiced. For some speech sounds the vocal cords do not vibrate, but remain open. Such sounds are said to be voiceless, and they arise from turbulence at a constriction of the vocal tract above the glottis (e.g., /s/ as in 'sit').

The speech sounds produced by a constriction are classified into a number of different types. A fricative consonant is characterised by a turbulent noise, and may consist of that noise alone (as in /s/), or may consist of that noise together with a glottal source (/z/). Stop con-

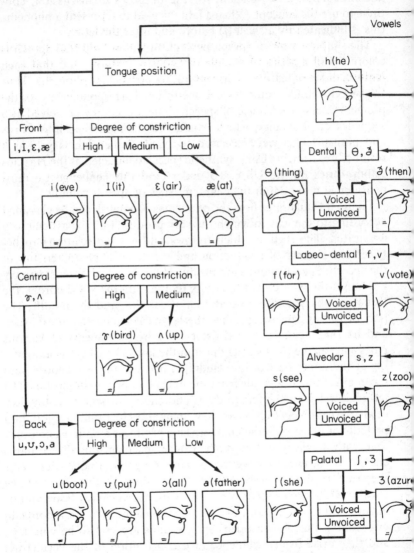

* In the above classification /e/ (hate), /o/ (obey) are considered as diphthongs and /tʃ/ (chew) and /dʒ/ (jar) are considered as stop-fricative combinations

Figure 6.1   Classification of phonemes according to their manner and

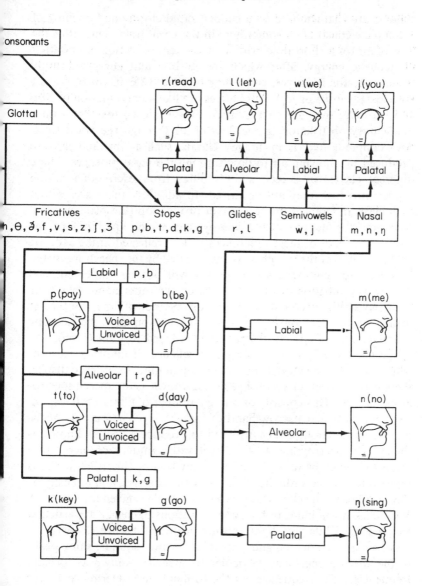

oduction. Adapted from figures in Potter, Kopp and Green (1947).

sonants are characterised by a sudden rapid closing and opening of a complete constriction somewhere in the vocal tract. This stops the flow of air for a short time, with a consequent reduction or cessation of acoustic energy, after which the airflow and energy abruptly resume. As for fricatives, stops may be voiced (as in /p/ or /b/) or voiceless (as in /t/ or /d/). Affricatives are like a combination of stop and fricative; they are characterised by turbulence together with a momentary obstruction to the flow of air through the vocal tract. An example is /dʒ/ as in 'judge'. Nasals, such as /m/ and /n/, are produced by allowing air to flow through the nasal passages. These different classes of speech sounds differ from each other in the *manner* in which they are produced. In addition, there are, within each class, differences in the *place* of production (the place where a constriction generates sound energy, e.g. teeth, lips, roof of the mouth, etc.). All of these differences will be reflected in the acoustic characteristics of the speech wave, as revealed by the speech spectrum. However, for consonants the spectra will not be static, but will change as a function of time. Vowels, on the other hand, may have relatively stable spectra, at least for short periods of time. For further details of the relationship between articulation and the acoustic characteristics of speech, the reader is referred to Fant (1960).

Speech, then, is an example par excellence of auditory patterns which vary in frequency, in amplitude and in time. In order to display these variations simultaneously a device known as the speech spectrograph is used. This consists of a large number of filters, each responsive to a particular narrow band of frequencies. The outputs of the filters as a function of time are used to produce a display known as the speech spectrogram. In this display the amount of energy in a given frequency band is plotted as a function of time. Frequency is represented on the ordinate, time along the abscissa, and intensity by the darkness of the line used. A typical example is given inFigure 6.2. Very dark areas indicate high concentrations of energy at particular frequencies, while very light areas indicate an absence of energy.

Many speech sounds, and particularly vowel sounds, show peaks in the spectral energy at particular frequencies, known as formant frequencies. The frequencies of the formants are determined by the shape of the vocal tract, which behaves as a filter modifying the glottal source. The formants are numbered, the one with the lowest frequency being called the first formant, the next the second, and so on. Vowel sounds may be characterised in terms of their formant

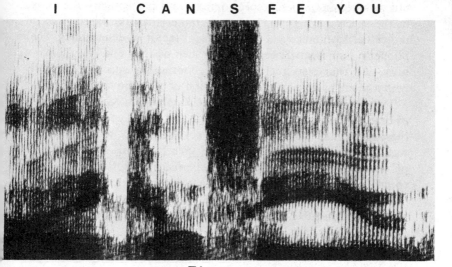

Figure 6.2 A speech spectrogram for the utterance 'I can see you'. Notice the concentration of energy at particular frequencies (formants), except for the /s/ sound, and the lack of silent intervals between successive words. The vertical striations correspond to individual periods of vocal cord vibration, and their spacing depends on the rate of this vibration.

frequencies and the amount of energy at each of these formants. As many as six formants may be observed in a speech spectrogram, but the first three are the most important for the purpose of identifying the vowel. There are, of course, other ways of analysing vowel sounds, as we saw in Chapter 4 (cf. the dimensional analysis approach by Plomp and his colleagues), but analysis in terms of formants has been by far the most common and most influential technique.

A marked characteristic of speech sounds is that there are often rapid changes in the frequency of a given formant or set of formants. These changes, known as formant transitions, have been found to be important acoustic cues for the perception of consonants. Speech sounds may be either periodic (voiced), in which case they will have a pitch, or noise-like (voiceless), in which case there will be no well-defined pitch, although timbre variations, based on frequency spectrum, may occur. Vowels, and some consonants, are periodic, and will be similar to the complex tones discussed in Chapter 4. Although they are composed of harmonics, the individual harmonics are usually

217

not resolved in a speech spectrogram, and perceptually the peaks in the spectral envelope (formants) rather than the frequencies of individual harmonics are the important factor in determining what phoneme is present. Speech sounds such as the 's' in 'hiss' have a noise-like character and display a continuous spectrum, usually with a much more uniform distribution of energy over frequency.

The speech spectrogram of a complete sentence may show a number of time intervals where there is little or no spectral energy. However, these silent intervals do not always correspond to 'spaces' between words, but often occur during the speech sounds representing a particular word. Thus in explaining speech perception we have to specify not only how the acoustic elements in the speech sound are 'decoded' into individual phonemes, but also how the sequence of sounds is segmented into individual words and syllables.

6.3 SPEECH PERCEPTION—THE CASE FOR A SPEECH MODE

In what is now a classic paper Liberman *et al.* (1967) gave a number of reasons for thinking that phonemes not only *were* not but *could* not be efficiently communicated by sounds that stand in a one-to-one correspondence with the phonemes. One of their arguments concerned the rate at which speech sounds occur. In rapid speech as many as 30 phonemes per second may occur, and it was argued that this would be too fast for resolution in the auditory system; the sounds would merge into an unanalysable buzz. We saw in Chapter 4 that listeners can, in fact, learn to identify sequences of sounds when the individual items are as short as 10 ms (corresponding to a rate of 100 items per second), but that at these short durations the listeners do not perceive each successive item separately but rather learn the overall sound pattern. It is likely that for continuous speech something similar applies. Even if there are acoustic cues in a one-to-one correspondence with the phonemes, these cues will not be perceived as discrete acoustic events. Rather the listener will recognise the sound pattern corresponding to a group of phonemes, such as those corresponding to a whole syllable, or even a word.

One of the most important arguments of Liberman *et al.* concerned the nature of the acoustic cues which underly the perception of particular phonemes. They used as an example the phoneme /d/ as in 'dawn'. A major cue for the perception of /d/ is a transition in the second formant. Indeed, Liberman *et al.* suggested that the

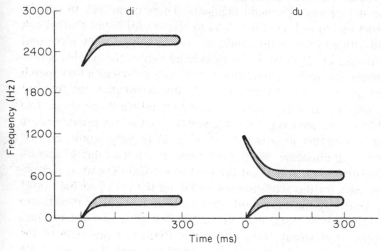

Figure 6.3 Highly simplified spectrographic patterns which are perceived as /di/ and /du/ when they are converted into sound. From Liberman *et al.* (1967), by permission of the authors and the American Psychological Association.

second formant transition was a major cue for most consonant sounds, and was 'probably the single most important carrier of linguistic information in the speech signal'. Consider the highly simplified spectrographic pattern shown in Figure 6.3. When these are converted into sound, the first formant transition (the change in frequency of the lowest formant at the beginning of the sound) provides a cue for the class of voiced stops /b, d, g/. Some other aspect of the sounds determines which of these three is actually heard. The sounds illustrated are actually identified as /di/ and /du/ when presented to listeners. On the basis of a number of perceptual experiments using such synthetic speech sounds, Liberman *et al.* concluded that the second formant transitions in the patterns are the cues for the perception of /d/ as opposed to /b/ or /g/. Notice that although listeners identify each of these sounds as beginning with the phoneme /d/, the acoustic cues at the beginning of the sounds are vastly different for the two examples presented. In the case of /di/ the transition rises from about 2200 to 2600 Hz; in /du/ it falls from 1200 to 700 Hz. Thus the same phoneme can be cued, in different contexts, by acoustic features that are vastly different.

A related argument concerns the non-existence of clear boundaries between successive phonetic segments. There is no way to cut the patterns shown in Figure 6.3 so as to recover /d/ segments that can be substituted one for the other, or even to obtain some piece that will sound like /d/ alone. If the right-hand half of the syllable is progressively removed, we hear either /d/ plus a vowel, or a non-speech sound. According to Liberman *et al.*, this is because 'the formant transition is, at every instant, providing information about two phonemes, the consonant and the vowel—that is, the phonemes are being transmitted in parallel'. An alternative view would be that since the /d/ phoneme cannot exist alone, it is not a 'unit' of speech.

Liberman *et al.* argue that the kind of context-dependent restructuring seen for the acoustic cues signalling the /d/ phoneme occurs quite generally for consonant sounds. Thus it is rarely possible to find invariant acoustic cues corresponding to a given consonant phoneme. For steady state vowels the frequency positions of the formants do provide more or less invariant cues, but vowels are rarely steady state in normal speech. Usually vowels are articulated between consonants at rather rapid rates, so that 'vowels also show substantial restructuring—that is, the acoustic signal at no point corresponds to the vowel alone, but rather shows, at any instant, the merged influences of the preceding or following consonant'. The general conclusion is that a single acoustic cue may carry information in parallel about successive phonemes. This reduces the rate at which discrete sounds must be perceived, but at the expense of a complex relation between cue and phoneme. Phoneme perception therefore requires a special decoder. Liberman *et al.* refer to those phonemes whose acoustic cues show considerable context-dependent restructuring as 'encoded', while those phonemes for which there are relatively invariant acoustic cues are called 'unencoded'. They suggested that the perception of encoded phonemes should differ from the perception of unencoded phonemes and from the perception of non-speech sounds.

One piece of evidence for a special 'speech mode' in auditory perception is the phenomenon of categorical perception. For an acoustic signal varying along a single dimension, such as frequency, we are normally able to discriminate many more stimuli than we can identify absolutely (see the section on auditory pattern perception in Chapter 4). However, for encoded phonemes it is found that listeners discriminate very little better than they can identify absolutely. Changes in the acoustic signal which do not change the phoneme identity are perceived with difficulty, or not at all, by the subject, while those acoustic changes which produce a change in phoneme identity are, of course, easily discriminated. Consider, for example, some simplified synthetic speech signals in which the second-formant transition is varied in relatively small, acoustically equal steps through a range sufficient to produce the three phonemes /b/, /d/ and /g/. One does not hear a series of small changes in the acoustic signal, but 'essentially quantal jumps from one perceptual category to another' (Liberman *et al.*, 1967). Thus we do not hear changes within one phoneme category, but only changes from one phoneme to another. This is called categorical perception. In order to demonstrate categorical perception both identification and discrimination tasks must be performed. The identification task establishes the boundaries between phonetic categories. The discrimination task is usually of the ABX type. Three successive stimuli are presented, and the listener is required to state whether the last stimulus is the same as the first or the second. For the ideal case of categorical perception discrimination would be high across category boundaries, but would drop to chance level for pairs of stimuli falling within one category. In practice the situation is rarely as straightforward as we have described here, but whenever discrimination of acoustic changes is good across phoneme boundaries and poor within phoneme categories, this is taken as evidence of categorical perception.

The situation with steady state vowels is very different. Small physical changes in the acoustic stimulus are perceived as such, so that one vowel may be heard to shade into another, and many intraphonemic variations are heard. Liberman *et al.* suggest that this is because vowels are much less encoded than speech sounds, so that they may be perceived in the same manner as non-speech sounds. However, vowel sounds in rapidly articulated speech do show restructuring, and there is evidence (Stevens, 1968) that perception of certain vowels in their proper dynamic context is more nearly categorical than is found for steady state vowels.

Although categorical perception has been considered to reflect the operation of a special speech decoder, there is some evidence that categorical perception can occur in a non-linguistic mode. Locke and Kellar (1973) obtained identification and discrimination functions for triads consisting of three simultaneous pure tones, using both musicians and non-musicians as subjects. Of the three tones in the triad, only the middle tone was varied, in small steps over a range sufficient to produce a chord of A minor (440, 523 and 659 Hz) at one end of the range, and a chord of A major (440, 554 and 659 Hz) at the other end. Categorisation was considerably more prominent among the musicians; they tended to recognise the triads as either A minor or A major. Further, the discrimination curves for musicians did parallel predictions from categorisation more closely than did the curves for non-musicians. In other words, the discrimination performance of musicians was better for frequency changes which altered the identity of the chord.

A second example of categorical perception in a non-linguistic mode is provided by the work of Cutting and Rosner (1974). They used as stimuli saw-tooth waves, generated by a Moog synthesiser, whose rise time was varied from 0 to 80 ms. The rapid-onset waves sound like a plucked string (guitar), while the slow-onset waves sound like a bowed string. Subjects were required to identify the stimuli (pluck or bow) and to discriminate them in an ABX paradigm. They found that there was a boundary in the identification functions at a rise time of 40–50 ms and that discrimination was good across the boundary but poor within a category.

The categorical perception observed in these experiments may indicate that the phenomenon depends in part on the ability to make an absolute identification of familiar auditory patterns rather than on the operation of a special speech decoder. This point will be discussed further later in the chapter.

A different line of evidence indicating that speech perception is different from the perception of non-speech is provided by studies establishing the regions in the brain that play a role in the perception of speech and non-speech sounds. These studies are based on the assumption that the crossed neural pathways from the ear to the brain (i.e. from the right ear to the left cerebral cortex, and vice versa) are generally more effective than the uncrossed pathways. If competing stimuli are presented simultaneously to the two ears (e.g. two different spoken messages), then speech stimuli presented to the right ear are better identified than those presented to the left, while the reverse is true for melodies (Broadbent and Gregory, 1964; Kimura, 1964). This suggests that encoded speech signals are more readily decoded in the left cerebral hemisphere than in the right. Studies of deficiencies in speech perception and production for people with brain lesions have also indicated that the left hemisphere plays a primary role in speech perception (Kimura, 1961).

A third line of evidence is provided by studies of the perception and identification of sounds which vary in the extent to which their acoustic characteristics approach those of speech. House *et al.* (1962) required subjects to learn to associate members of various ensembles of acoustic stimuli with buttons on a response box. They found that stimuli with spectral and temporal properties similar to those of speech are not learned more readily than simpler stimuli unless they are actually identified by the listener as speech. Thus, as Stevens and House (1972) have put it, '. . . although one can imagine an acoustic continuum in which the sounds bear a closer and closer relation to speech, there is no such continuum as far as the perception of the sounds is concerned—the perception is dichotomous. Sounds are perceived either as linguistic or as nonlinguistic entities.'

Overall, then, the evidence for some special kind of speech-processing mechanism is quite strong. We tend to perceive speech sound categorically, so that most speech sounds are perceived as having a particular identity, and not as being 'in between' two classes of speech sound. There is good evidence that particular parts of the brain are specialised for dealing with speech. And when we are presented with speech-like sounds, there is a perceptual dichotomy: either the sounds are perceived as speech or they are not. Stevens and House (1972) suggested that 'the listener need not be set for speech prior to his hearing the signal; his prepared state is triggered by the presence of a signal that has appropriate acoustic properties'. Very probably there is a strong involuntary component to this 'triggering' of the speech mode; no matter how hard we try, it is impossible to hear speech in terms of its acoustical characteristics, i.e. as a series of hisses, whistles, buzzes, etc. Rather we perceive a unified stream of speech sounds.

6.4 MODELS OF SPEECH PERCEPTION

There are no models of speech perception that are sufficiently accurately specified to allow rigorous experimental testing, but two theoretical approaches have had a considerable influence on the direction and emphasis of research in speech perception. These two approaches are those of the Haskins Laboratory investigators and of Stevens and his colleagues at the Massachusetts Institute of Technology. Both groups have been strongly influenced by the problem of the complex relationship between acoustic cues and perceived phonemic segments and by the problem of segmenting the speech wave into syllables and words.

The approach of the Haskins group has been called the 'motor theory' of speech perception. They proposed that speech perception requires a special decoding mechanism which proceeds by reference to articulatory processes. The basic idea is that somewhere in the nervous system the neural signals corresponding to the sensory input are brought into correspondence with internally generated neural signals which would have produced the articulatory movements leading to that sensory input. Early versions of this model, such as that presented by Liberman (1957), assumed that the patterns generated by the listener were actually produced as covert articulatory responses, whose proprioceptive feedback was compared with the stored speech sound. In later versions this viewpoint has been somewhat modified, since there is clear evidence that speech may be perceived in the absence of any measurable articulatory response on the part of the listener. Thus Liberman *et al.* (1963) suggested that 'the neural commands themselves, or rather their equivalents in the central nervous system, might be used to provide the reference system in terms of which the decoding (of speech) is carried out'.

Notice that the emphasis is on an active process of speech recognition rather than on a passive registration of the acoustic stimulus and its direct translation into speech. Liberman *et al.* (1967) set forward a number of reasons for believing that speech perception proceeds via production rather than via a straightforward auditory decoder.

Firstly, they suggested that since the listener is also a speaker, '. . . it seems unparsimonious to assume that the speaker-listener employs two entirely separate processes of equal status, one for encoding language and the other for decoding it. A simpler assumption is that there is only one process, with appropriate linkages between sensory and motor components.' This argument is somewhat dubious since a passive theorist might argue that the processes involved in the motor theory approach are excessively complex and unwieldy, and would result in an inherently slow mechanism. Further, it is not at all clear how the patterns of neural activity corresponding to articulatory commands would be transformed so that they could be compared with the neural traces corresponding to the stored speech signal. Such a transformation would have to take into account all of the complex processing of the auditory stimulus which occurs in the peripheral auditory system, and we have seen that for a wide-band signal this is by no means simple.

A second argument of Liberman *et al.* derives from observations of electromyographic (EMG) signals from the speech musculature. These have led to the conclusion that the perceptions of a listener in response to speech are more closely related to the patterns of articulation that produce those speech signals than to the acoustic signals themselves. Thus the patterns of muscular movement which produce a given speech sound may lie more nearly in a one-to-one correspondence with the perception of that sound than the acoustic signals. Again, however, this does not necessarily favour a motor theory. It may well be the case that when a speaker 'decides' to say a particular speech sound, the neural commands corresponding to that sound are more or less invariant. The fact that the acoustic consequences of those neural commands are not invariant is merely a result of the particular way that the articulatory apparatus works. Thus the higher correlation between production and perception than between acoustic signals and perception does not necessarily imply the mediation of production in perception. It merely reflects the fact that the acoustic consequences of a sequence of muscular movements vary according to the order in which those movements are strung together.

The theoretical approach of Stevens and his colleagues is similar in spirit to that of the Haskins group, but is considerably more specific. It has been called the analysis by synthesis model. According to this model, the peripheral patterns of neural activity corresponding to speech sounds are subject to a preliminary analysis, and are also held in a temporary store. Sometimes this preliminary analysis provides sufficient information for phonetic information to be passed on immediately to higher levels of processing. Often, however, the analysis is insufficient, in which case the listener makes a hypothesis as to the nature of the speech sounds. This hypothesis allows the listener to generate patterns, either at the muscular level or at the neural level, corresponding to the articulations which would actually be necessary to produce the hypothesised sounds. These patterns can then be compared with the patterns in the temporary store. The comparison either confirms that the hypothesised utterance is correct or generates an error message which can be used as the basis for further hypotheses. Provided that the error message carries useful new information, no more than two or three hypotheses will be necessary before the utterance is 'correctly' perceived. Notice that this model requires that there be at least a few invariant cues, so that a reasonable initial hypothesis can be generated, otherwise an infinity of bad guesses might result. We may consider the analysis by synthesis model as a more detailed and slightly modified form of the motor theory suggested by the Haskins group. Just as for the motor theory, a major problem for the model is to explain how the two types of patterns could be compared. The generated pattern is a set of neural commands which if executed would result in the articulation of a particular phoneme or word. The stored pattern is some kind of neural representation or memory trace corresponding to the acoustic pattern. Clearly, some very complex transformations would be necessary before any comparison could occur.

One of the strongest arguments in favour of 'active' theories of speech perception was their ability to explain the phenomenon of categorical perception, although, as we shall see, other explanations have now emerged. As we described earlier, the perception of certain speech sounds is discontinuous, even when the acoustic signal is varied continuously. It turns out that the corresponding articulations are also discontinuous. Consider an example given by Liberman *et al.* (1967): 'With /b, d, g/, we can vary the acoustic cue along a continuum, which corresponds, in effect, to closing the vocal tract at various points along its length. But in actual speech the closing is accomplished by discontinuous or categorically different gestures: by the lips for /b/, the tip of the tongue for /d/, and the back of the tongue for /g/.' Thus the categorical perception of these speech sounds can be explained by assuming that they are decoded with reference to articulation and that the articulation is itself categorical.

Once again, however, it is not clear that this is the appropriate explanation of categorical perception. Firstly, there is evidence that non-speech sounds may be perceived categorically (see the experiments by Locke and Kellar, 1973, and Cutting and Rosner, 1974, described earlier in this chapter, and the discussion by Lane, 1965). Secondly, an alternative hypothesis has emerged which explains the data in a more satisfactory way: that the differences in perception which are observed for 'encoded' consonants and relatively 'unencoded' vowels may be explained in terms of differences in the extent to which the acoustic cues can be retained in acoustic memory (see below, and also Darwin and Baddeley, 1974 and Pisoni, 1973). The acoustic cues corresponding to the consonant parts of speech sounds are generally at a much lower intensity than those for vowel sounds. In addition, the cues for consonants fluctuate more rapidly and last for a shorter time than those for vowels. Consequently, the acoustic cues for consonants will be much more ephemeral in acoustic memory. It may be that by the time these acoustic cues have been processed in the identification of the phoneme they are lost from auditory memory. Thus further discimination, within phoneme categories, will not be possible. However, for speech sounds such as vowels, the acoustic cues will be retained in acoustic memory for longer periods of time, so that additional discriminations, based upon these stored cues, can be made. As was mentioned earlier (see Section 6.3), the triggering of the 'speech mode' is probably involuntary. Thus the initial processing of cues in acoustic memory, when we are presented with speech sounds, will always relate to the linguistic properties of those sounds. It is only after this initial analysis that discrimination of the cues in a non-linguistic mode is possible. Those cues which are efficiently stored in acoustic memory will then give rise to continuous perception, whereas if the cues corresponding to a given phoneme are lost, only discrimination based on the prior categorisation will be possible. We should note that the ABX design used to test for categorical perception inevitably confounds perception with memory.

In summary, the arguments put forward by Liberman *et al.* (1967) in favour of a motor theory approach can be interpreted in other ways. Although the evidence for a special mode of speech perception is quite strong, the evidence that this special mode operates by reference to articulation is weak. Indeed, a number of workers have presented arguments against a motor theory approach. For example, Fant (1973) says: 'The alternative view I would like to propose here that if the auditory analysis in the hearing process has proceeded so far as to allow the proposed articulatory matching, the decoding could proceed without an articulatory reference.' Perhaps one of the most crucial pieces of evidence has been presented by Lenneberg (1962). He described the case of a patient who had an organic defect which prevented the acquisition of the motor skill necessary for speaking a language. Nevertheless, the patient could understand speech and possessed all the grammatical skills necessary for a complete understanding of language. Here, then, is a clear case of someone who cannot speak, but can understand speech. Of course, modern versions of the motor theory assume that mediation takes

15-2

place not via articulations themselves, but via the neural commands corresponding to those articulations. Thus, in theory, it is not necessary for a listener to speak in order to understand speech. However, it is difficult to understand how a person who had *never* spoken could learn to associate speech sounds with the appropriate neural commands. Similar cases have been reported by Fourcin (1975).

Although we have been arguing that speech perception need not operate by reference to articulation, this does not mean that the listener perceives speech via the passive registration of individual acoustic features. On the contrary, it is likely that the listener not only sets up hypotheses concerning speech signals already received, but also makes predictions about what speech signals will occur next. If a given speech element is exceedingly probable in the context of the utterance as a whole, then that element will be 'heard' when the acoustic cues are minimal or even completely absent. Even for words spoken in isolation, factors related to word probability may affect recognition especially under noisy listening conditions. Broadbent (1967) reported that common words tend to be detected at lower signal-to-noise ratios than rare words, or to be detected more often at the same signal-to-noise ratio. He called this the word-frequency effect, and discussed four models to explain the effect. He concluded in favour of a model based on signal detection theory (see Section 3.7), which has been proposed and elaborated by Morton (1964). According to this model, a listener has an internal 'dictionary' of word units, such that when a unit is caused to be fired, a word corresponding to that unit is perceived. Two separate factors determine whether or not a given unit will fire. The first factor is the sensory evidence relating to the acoustic features specifying the word. The second factor is the response bias of the unit—a measure of its 'readiness' to fire—which will be affected by such factors as word probability and context. Thus the dictionary unit corresponding to a given word will fire on the basis of less sensory evidence when that word is highly probable, either because of context or because it is a common word.

This model accounts well for the influence of non-acoustic factors in speech perception, and it would be capable of rapid operation: a dictionary unit would fire 'automatically' on presentation of the appropriate sensory evidence, provided that the sensory evidence were sufficient to exceed the threshold of the unit at that time. However, the model is inadequate in many respects. It does not say how the sensory evidence would be processed in extracting acoustic features indicative of any particular word. In other words, the problem of non-invariance between acoustic cue and perceived phoneme remains. We should note that this problem persists even if units of greater length, such as the syllable or word, are considered. Further, the system does not allow for a re-analysis of the sensory data if the 'wrong' dictionary unit fires. Sub-threshold excitation of other dictionary units does not result in any output from the system. Finally, the output of the system is in terms of the identity of words and not in terms of their perceptual attributes. Thus it is not clear how these attributes (man's voice or woman's, accent, direction of sound, loudness, etc.) would be linked to the outputs of the dictionary unit system. This could be a serious problem in situations where several people are talking at once.

Recently it has been suggested that the role of encoded or overlapping cues in speech perception has been somewhat overemphasised (Fischer-Jørgensen, 1972). Cole and Scott (1974) have noted that speech perception involves the simultaneous identification of at least three qualitatively different types of cues: invariant cues, context-dependent cues (e.g. frequency transitions) and cues provided by the waveform envelope. In a review of the literature on consonant phonemes—traditionally considered as highly encoded speech sounds—Cole and Scott conclude that *all* consonant phonemes are accompanied by invariant features, i.e. by acoustic cues which accompany a particular phoneme in any vowel environment. In some cases the invariant information is sufficient uniquely to define the consonant, while in other cases the invariant features limit perception to a possible pair or triplet of phonemes. They show, further, that transitional cues are also present in all consonant–vowel syllables. In other words, any given syllable contains both invariant and transitional cues. The transitional information may sometimes be necessary to discriminate between a pair of phonemes which have been signalled by invariant cues.

Cole and Scott concluded that 'the major source of information about the identity of consonant phonemes during speech perception is provided by invariant cues'. Many workers in this area would disagree with this rather strong conclusion. While it is possible to find a number of relatively invariant cues for consonants in single words or syllables articulated clearly in isolation, these cues are rarely so apparent in rapid connected speech. In many cases there are a number of separate cues associated with a given phoneme, and the relative importance of these cues will vary according to the context. In addition, the effective use of many cues has been shown to depend upon information obtained from previous portions of the same utterance, such as the rate of speech or the size of the vocal tract of the speaker (which influences the values of formant frequencies corresponding to any given phoneme). Thus it seems certain that for most real speech situations, which may involve background noises and sloppy articulations, the listener has to perform a fairly complex decoding process in order to make optimal use of the available information.

Although there is some debate about the relative importance of encoded and invariant cues in phoneme identification, it is clear that encoded or transitional cues are of considerable importance in speech perception. Indeed, speech from which all transitions have been removed is extremely difficult to understand, and sounds very unnatural. Liberman *et al.* (1967) have argued that the transitional cues provide the listener with important information about the serial order of speech sounds. For example, the transitional cues for /da/ and /ad/ are 'mirror images' (in time) of one another. Thus a falling second formant tells the listener that the /d/ was before the /a/, whereas a rising second formant tells him the opposite. Cole and Scott have suggested another role of transitions—that of maintaining the speech wave as an integrated perceptual whole. We saw in Chapter 4 that a series of alternating high and low tones tends to split, perceptually, into two separate auditory streams. Bregman and Campbell (1971) called this primary auditory stream segregation. This particular phenomenon seems to be part of a more general tendency of the auditory system to group stimuli according to their physical characteristics (Broadbent, 1958). If this is the case, it is difficult, at first sight, to understand why speech does not also split into a number of separate streams, composed of, say, high-frequency bursts of noise, high-frequency periodic energy and low-frequency periodic energy. The answer may lie, according to Cole and Scott, in the role of the transitional cues.

We saw in Chapter 4 that stream segregation for sequences of tones is reduced by connecting high- and low-frequency tones with frequency glides (Bregman and Dannenbring, 1973). Frequency transitions in speech sounds may play a similar role in reducing stream segregation. Certain consonant–vowel syllables are composed of an initial invariant portion, often of a noise-like character, followed by transitions and a vowel. If the initial invariant portion is removed, leaving only the transition and the vowel, then the perception changes so that a stop consonant (e.g. /ba/ or /da/) is heard. For example, if the invariant portion is removed from either /fa/, /va/ or /ma/, then the syllable /ba/ is heard in each case, because each of these syllables has similar transitional cues: /f/, /v/ and /m/ all have the same place of articulation.

Cole and Scott reasoned that repeated presentations of a single syllable might result in auditory stream segregation, so that 'the invariant energy should group with its own prior and subsequent repetitions to form one perceptual stream, while subjects should hear the embedded stop consonant syllable in a separate stream'. Using tape loops, they presented single consonant–vowel syllables to subjects at the rate of two repetitions per second, and found exactly the predicted results: '. . . a syllable such as /sa/ was heard to segregate into "hissing noise plus /da/"', while a syllable such as /fa/ was heard as a "cat hiss plus /ba/" '. In order to investigate the effect of the transitions upon this stream segregation, Cole and Scott used syllables in which the transitions were removed, so that the consonant noise was spliced directly onto the steady state vowel. This did not affect syllable recognition for single presentations, but when these transitionless syllables were presented repeatedly on a tape loop, the subjects reported a segregation of the stimulus into consonant noise and the vowel /a/. This in itself is not surprising, but it is noteworthy that segregation for the transitionless vowels occurred after only three or four repetitions, whereas normal syllables required 60 or more repetitions. Thus it seems that transitions play a major role in inhibiting the perceptual segregation of consonant noise and the periodic vowel sound.

It is likely that a number of other factors play a role in maintaining the speech wave as an integrated perceptual whole. One of these was mentioned earlier in this chapter. For rapid speech it seems likely that we do not perceive each phoneme separately, but rather that we recognise the sound pattern corresponding to a group of phonemes, such as those which compose a complete word or syllable. Any such group of phonemes is likely to have several features in common with preceding and following groups of phonemes (each is likely to contain both noise-like and periodic sounds, and there would probably be some overlap of frequency components), so that stream segregation between the groups would be unlikely to occur. In addition, speech contains stress and intonation patterns which may extend over several successive words, and these patterns may serve as links between successive elements in the speech wave, thus maintaining an integrated perceptual stream.

So far our discussion of the physical characteristics of speech has been almost exclusively concerned with the patterns revealed by the speech spectrogram, i.e. with variations in sound spectrum as a function of time. This type of analysis has been exceedingly influential, one of the main reasons being that, to a first approximation, a similar kind of analysis appears to take place in the auditory system. Thus the search for invariant acoustic cues corresponding to particular phonemes has mainly been directed towards finding such cues in the speech spectrogram. There is, however, another way of describing the speech wave which is physically and conceptually simpler than the speech spectrogram, and which does appear to have a good deal of perceptual relevance—namely the waveform envelope.

Imagine that we plot the speech waveform in terms of pressure variations as a function of time. Such a plot could be obtained as a display on an oscilloscope if the pressure variations were converted into voltage variations by means of a microphone. The envelope is the curve produced by drawing a smooth line passing through the peaks in the waveform; it is a kind of 'outline' of the waveform. A typical example is given in Figure 6.4, for the utterance 'I'm a waveform'. Notice that for much of the time the envelope shows peaks which are fairly regularly spaced. This indicates that the speech sounds are periodic and involve the vibration of the vocal cords (i.e. they are voiced sounds). The time intervals between these peaks in the envelope are the same as the correponding periods of vibration for the vocal cords. The part of the envelope corresponding to the 've' in wave and the 'f' in form does not show these periodic peaks, because of the noise-like nature of these sounds, and it also has a lower amplitude. Variations in amplitude, and therefore in loudness, also occur during the voiced parts of the speech.

Clearly, then, the waveform envelope gives us information about fluctuations in amplitude as a function of time. Both amplitude and duration have been demonstrated to be of considerable importance in determining the so-called prosodic features of speech (those concerned with intonation, stress, etc.). Even a period of silence can provide cues for stress, enabling us to distinguish between such

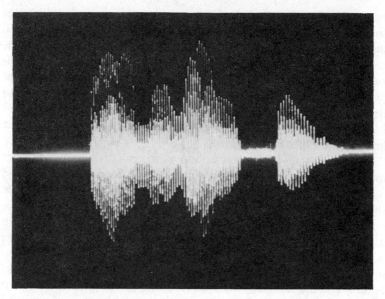

Figure 6.4 A photograph of an oscilloscope display showing the envelope of the utterance 'I'm a waveform'.

phrases as 'lighthouse keeper' and 'light housekeeper'. However, such cues are only useful if they are evaluated in relation to duration and amplitude cues from adjacent syllables; speech rates and average intensities vary considerably, so that a measurement of amplitude or duration taken in isolation would have little significance. Thus our use of amplitude and duration cues in determining prosodic features indicates that information relating to the waveform envelope can be retained in storage for relatively long time periods.

There is good evidence that the waveform envelope also provides information about the phonemic composition of speech. Many experiments have shown that features such as duration, short periods of silence, relative amplitude and pitch can influence the perception of particular phonemes. All of these features can be extracted from the waveform envelope. An indication of the amount of information which may be carried in the waveform envelope is provided by an experiment of Katz and Berry (1971). They imposed upon a white noise 'carrier' the waveform envelopes of various speech stimuli. They found quite good intelligibility scores for this 'speech-modulated' white noise, although words in sentences were discriminated better than words in isolation, and vowels were discriminated better than consonants. Thus to some extent the auditory system is able to decode speech stimuli on the basis of time–amplitude variations alone. The ability to extract information from the waveform envelope is not, of course, unique to speech; we saw in Chapter 4 that periodically interrupted white noise has a pitch corresponding to the envelope repetition rate, and in Chapter 5 that the envelope of high-frequency amplitude-modulated tones can be used in the lateralisation of such sounds.

It is clear that in the perception of speech the human listener makes use of a great variety of types of information which are available in the speech wave. Many different cues may be available to signal a given speech element (phoneme), but the cues may not be constant and may differ in relative importance from utterance to utterance. Thus many kinds of context-dependent variations in the acoustic cues occur, and accurate speech recognition will depend upon the listener's ability to allow for the context and compute its effects. The multidimensional nature of the acoustic cues allows for a high level of redundancy in the speech wave; there may be several different acoustic cues for a given phoneme, of which just one or two might be sufficient for recognition. This redundancy can be used to overcome the ambiguities inherent in the speech, to lessen the effects of interfering stimuli, to compensate for distortions in the signal (for example, when the speech is transmitted over a telephone line), and to allow for poor articulation on the part of the speaker. At a higher level, errors made in identifying a speech sound from its acoustic pattern can be corrected by the listener's knowledge of the kinds of speech signals which can be produced by the human vocal tract, by reference to linguistic rules, by the 'sense' of the message, and by knowledge of the characteristics of the speaker, e.g. accent or sex.

6.5 THE RESISTANCE OF SPEECH TO CORRUPTING INFLUENCES

One way to assess the degree of redundancy in the speech wave is to eliminate or distort certain features and to determine the effect of this on the intelligibility of the speech. The results of such experiments have indicated that speech is, in fact, remarkably resistant to many kinds of quite severe distortions. Most of the experimental data have been obtained using articulation testing methods: a speaker reads a list of syllables, words or sentences to a listener, or group of listeners, and the percentage of itsems correctly recorded by the listener(s) is called the articulation score.

One factor which can affect speech intelligibility is the amount of background noise. For satisfactory communication the average speech level should exceed that of the noise by 6 dB (i.e. the S/N ratio should be $+6$ dB). When speech and noise levels are equal (0 dB S/N ratio), the word articulation score reaches about 50 per cent. However, speech may be intelligible at negative S/N ratios (where the speech level is below that of the noise) for connected speech, particularly if the listener is familiar with the subject matter, or if the speech and the noise come from different directions in space (this is an example of the BMLD phenomenon which was discussed in Chapter 5). In many practical situations the noise is intermittent rather than continuous. This decreases the effectiveness of the noise in masking the speech by an amount depending on the on–off ratio of the noise and the interruption rate. At high interruption rates (above about 200 per second) the noise has effects similar to those of continuous noise. At rates between 1 and 200 per second it is possible to patch together the bits of speech heard between the noise, so that the noise is not a very effective masker. At very slow interruption rates whole words or groups of words may be masked, while others are heard perfectly. Thus articulation scores drop once more.

A second factor which may affect speech intelligibility is a change in frequency spectrum. Many transmission systems (e.g. a telephone line) pass only a limited range of frequencies, and some of the first investigations of speech intelligibility were conducted by engineers of the Bell Telephone Laboratories, in an attempt to assess the importance of frequency range. This can be investigated using filters which pass only certain frequencies. A high-pass filter transmits all frequency components whose frequencies are above a certain cut-off frequency, while a low-pass filter transmits all frequencies below a certain cut-off frequency. A band-pass filter has both upper and lower cut-off frequencies, and transmits only those frequency components whose frequencies lie between the two (see Figure 1.4). Experiments using such filters, with variable cut-off frequencies, have shown that no particular frequency components are essential for speech recognition. For example, if all frequency components above 1800 Hz are filtered out, using a low-pass filter, then the syllable articulation score is about 67 per cent, while normal conversation is fully intelligible. However, speech is equally intelligible if instead we use a high-pass filter to remove all frequency components below 1800 Hz. Experiments using band-pass filters have shown that, over a fairly wide range of centre frequencies, a surprisingly narrow band of frequencies is sufficient for satisfactory recognition. For example, a band of frequencies from 1000 Hz to 2000 Hz is sufficient to give a sentence articulation score of about 90 per cent. Clearly, then, the information carried by the speech wave is not confined to any particular frequency range. This fits in very well with our notion of speech as a multidimensional stimulus, with many acoustic cues for any given phoneme.

A third kind of disrupting influence which commonly occurs is peak-clipping. If an amplifier or other part of a transmission system is overloaded, then the peaks of the waveform may be flattened off, or clipped. In severe cases the clipping level can be only 1 or 2 per cent of the original speech wave's peak values, with the result that the original speech wave, with its complex waveshape, is transformed into a series of rectangular pulses. This severe distortion does degrade the quality and naturalness of speech, but it has surprisingly little effect on intelligibility; word articulation scores of 80 or 90 per cent can still be obtained.

We see, then, that speech is intelligible under a wide variety of conditions where we might have expected rather poor performance. It remains intelligible in the presence of large amounts of background noise, or when we remove all but a small part of the speech spectrum, or when we destroy time–amplitude variations in the waveform by peak-clipping. Once again we are led to the conclusion that no single aspect of the speech wave is essential for speech perception. Thus the speech wave is highly redundant. Each of the disruptions which we have described will destroy some of the cues carried in the speech waveform, but the remaining cues are sufficient to convey the message. This is, of course, of great practical advantage. If speech perception depended on a near-perfect transmission of sound from speaker to listener, then speech communication in most real situations would become extremely difficult, and devices like the telephone would have to be much more elaborate and costly than they are. Nature has designed the speech communication process so that it can operate under a great variety of adverse conditions.

6.6 GENERAL CONCLUSIONS

We have seen that speech is a multidimensional stimulus varying in a complex way as a function of both frequency and time. Although the speech wave can be described in terms of amplitude and time, this does not seem to be the most appropriate description from the point of view of the auditory system. Neither is a description in terms of static spectra satisfactory. The representation which best fits the perceived nature of speech, and which is in accordance with the known functioning of the auditory system, uses the dimensions of intensity, frequency and time, as in the speech spectrogram. This shows how the short-term spectrum of the speech varies as a function of time.

A basic problem in the study of speech perception is to relate the properties of the speech wave to the linguistic units of which speech is composed. It is still not clear whether the basic unit of perception is the phoneme or the syllable. A description in terms of phonemes achieves a considerable economy in terms of the number of separate sound patterns which have to be analysed and remembered by the listener, since the number of phonemes is much less than the number of possible syllables. However, this type of economy may not be important in human perception. The ease and consistency with which the phonetician can describe an utterance in terms of phonemic units also argues for the phoneme as a unit of perception. On the other hand, for rapid connected speech the psychoacoustic evidence indicates that the individual phonemes would occur too rapidly to be separately perceived in correct temporal order. Thus the recognition of the overall sound pattern corresponding to a longer segment, such as a syllable, is indicated.

A related problem is that of finding acoustic cues in the speech waveform which would unambiguously signal a particular linguistic unit. Invariant relationships between acoustic cues and some phonemes have proved almost impossible to find, particularly for consonants. Thus, if the phoneme is the basic unit of perception, then decisions about phoneme identity must be taken with regard to information obtained over the whole syllable. In some cases a phoneme will only be correctly identified if information over a group of several words (giving information about the rate of speech, the size of the vocal tract of the speaker, etc.) is utilised. The complex relationship between the speech wave itself and the linguistic units of which speech is composed has been one of the central problems in speech perception, and has had a powerful influence on the development of theories of speech perception.

There is good evidence that speech is a special kind of auditory stimulus, and that speech stimuli are perceived and processed in a different way from non-speech stimuli. The evidence derives from studies of categorical perception, the phenomenon that speech sounds can be discriminated only when they are identified as being linguistically different; from studies of cerebral asymmetry, which indicate that certain parts of the brain are specialised for dealing with speech; and from the speech–non-speech dichotomy, the phenomenon that speech-like sounds are either perceived as speech or as something completely non-linguistic. Examples of this latter effect may occur when listening to faulty synthetic speech which only poorly approximates real speech. This will often be heard as a confusing mixture of buzzes, puffs of noise, whistles, etc., but the listener may suddenly switch into the 'speech mode' when the cacophony becomes intelligible speech.

The complex and variable relationship between the acoustic waveform and the phoneme has led to the development of a number of 'active' models of speech perception, in which speech is decoded by reference to articulatory processes. In one form of these models preliminary analysis of the speech wave, together with any available contextual information, is used to generate a hypothesis about the nature of the utterance. This hypothesised utterance is then checked against the stored neural representation of the speech signal, and if a match is achieved, then that utterance is perceived. In order for such a comparison to be possible, the stored speech and the hypothesised utterance must be transformed so that they are in comparable forms, which in itself would be a highly complex task. An inherent disadvantage of such a system is that in the absence of contextual cues it might be necessary to generate many different hypotheses before a satisfactory match was achieved, so that the process would be intrinsically slow. In fact, we can recognise words spoken in isolation rapidly and easily. At the present time there is no compelling evidence in favour of the active approaches, although it is generally accepted that speech perception involves decoding processes of considerable complexity.

It is clear that speech perception involves processing at many different levels and that separate information at each level may be used to resolve ambiguities or to correct errors which occur at other levels. The initial analysis of speech sounds into phonemes (or syllables) can be checked and readjusted by a stored knowledge of phonetic constraints, i.e. by a knowledge of the kinds of ways in which one phoneme can follow another. Our knowledge of syntactics (grammatical rules) and semantics (word meanings) allows further adjustments and corrections, while situational cues such as speaker identity and previous message content provide yet further information. It is quite possible that the processing of speech does not occur in a hierarchical way from one level to the next, but that there are extensive links between each level. Thus the information at any level may be reanalysed on the basis of information from other levels. Even some details of the speech wave itself may be retained for a short time in 'echoic memory' so that reanalyses may be made.

The multidimensional nature of speech sounds, and the large amount of independent information which is available at different levels of processing, produce a high level of redundancy in speech. This is reflected in the finding that speech intelligibility is relatively little affected by severe corrupting influences. Speech can be accurately understood in the presence of large amounts of background noise, or when it is severely altered by filtering, interruption or peak-clipping. Thus speech represents a highly efficient way of communicating under difficult conditions.

7

New Developments, Practical Applications and Future Outlook

7.1 INTRODUCTION

A large portion of this book has been concerned with the analysis of the basic sensory processes involved in the perception of stimuli such as tones, clicks and noises. To some extent this choice of subject matter is constrained by the history of research in auditory perception. The philosophy of workers in this area has been to use simple, reproducible stimuli in order to discover general rules which can then be applied to the more complex sounds which we encounter in everyday life. In many cases the results using these 'simple' stimuli have been so complex and intriguing that, in spite of considerable research effort, there is no general agreement as to the underlying mechanisms or as to how the results should be applied to more complex stimuli. However, this should not be taken to imply that the results are fruitless and that no useful general principles have emerged. Indeed, practically all the areas of research covered so far—loudness, masking, pitch, localisation and speech—have immediate counterparts in everyday life and have yielded useful applications. It is the purpose of this chapter to describe a few of the practical applications of auditory research and to suggest some possible future developments. In addition, some recently discovered auditory 'effects' will be described, not because of their immediate practical relevance, but because they may be important in understanding the way in which complex auditory stimuli are analysed.

7.2 ADAPTATION EFFECTS AND CHANNELS

In recent years a great deal of work on sensory systems has centred around the concept of 'channels' or groups of neurones responsive to particular properties of stimuli. This has been particularly true of the visual system, where there is evidence for channels 'tuned' to orientation, colour, spatial frequency, movement, and so on. The evidence for these channels comes from two quite separate sources, neurophysiological data and psychophysical data. As an example of the former, cells in the visual cortex have been found which respond best to lines of a particular orientation. The psychophysical evidence comes largely from studies of adaptation effects. The basic idea behind this has been well expressed by Mollon (1974): 'If one suspects that a particular attribute of the stimulus is subject to a specialised analysis, then the principle is to try to fatigue, or "adapt", selectively the neural mechanism tuned to detect that particular attribute.' This fatigue or adaptation will then be revealed as an after-effect of some kind, such as an elevation of threshold for the detection of that particular attribute of the stimulus.

In the auditory system one type of organisation by channels is well known and widely accepted, namely the tonotopic organisation; different neurones respond selectively to particular frequency components of stimuli, and any single neurone in the auditory nerve will respond optimally to only a relatively narrow range of frequencies. Thus it is quite common to use the phrase 'high-frequency channels' to refer to that group of neurones having high characteristic frequencies. However, at the level of the auditory cortex the tonotopic organisation appears to be much less well-defined, and many neurones will not respond to steady pure-tones at all (see Section 1.5). It is thus quite possible that cortical neurones are 'tuned' to more complex properties of stimuli than pure-tone frequency, and recent psychophysical evidence has tended to support this view. In the auditory cortex of the cat some neurones respond selectively to tones whose frequencies are changing in a particular direction or at a particular rate, or to tones which are modulated in frequency, so as to have a warbling quality (see Figure 3.4 for an illustration of the waveform of such sounds). Kay and Matthews (1972), using adaptation techniques, have presented evidence showing that channels tuned for the detection of such modulation may exist in the human auditory system. They presented an adapting tone whose frequency was sinusoidally modulated at a particular rate (say 8 times per second), and immediately after cessation of this stimulus they measured the ability to detect frequency modulation in a tone that was much more weakly modulated (i.e. in which the swing in frequency was not so great). They found that when the rate of modulation of the test tone was close to that of the adapting tone, the sensitivity was considerably reduced. The frequency deviation in the modulated test tone had to be increased to about three times the pre-exposure threshold to be detectable immediately after exposure to the adapting tone. Further, the effect was 'tuned' to modulation rate, so that when the modulation rate of the test tone was one-half or two times that of the adapting tone, the effect was very small. The effects were observed for modulation rates of the adapting tone from 1 per second up to 80 per second, although the largest effects occur around the middle of this range. Kay and Matthews showed that the adaptation did not depend critically on the adaptation and test tones having the same 'carrier' frequency, although this did have some effect. They showed, further, that the detectability of frequency modulation at a rate of 8 per second was not affected by prior exposure to a tone that was *amplitude*-modulated at a rate of 8 per second. Thus it is not simply the rhythm of the stimulus which is important. They concluded that the channels indicated by these experiments are not concerned with modulation periodicity *per se* or with signal spectrum or carrier frequency, but with instantaneous frequency changes. However, rate of frequency change cannot be the critical factor, since the rate of change of frequency (in Hz per second) is considerably different for the adapting stimulus and the test stimulus on which it has a maximal effect. It seems that the periodicity of the frequency changes is the crucial factor in adapting these channels, but the changes must be glides in frequency rather than instantaneous changes; the detectability of a sinusoidal modulation in frequency is not affected by prior exposure to a square-wave modulation (abrupt changes between one frequency and another).

Kay and Matthews (1972) suggested that these channels could be concerned with the extraction of certain features from speech signals, although it is not at all clear why channels with these particular characteristics should have evolved. It is the case that frequency changes are commonly observed in speech, but these changes are rarely of the periodic nature which these channels would require for activation. Other workers have attempted to investigate more directly the possibility that there are channels tuned for detecting particular features of speech sounds (Eimas and Corbit, 1973; Eimas, Cooper and Corbit, 1973; Bailey, 1973). These workers have exploited the phenomenon of categorical perception which occurs for

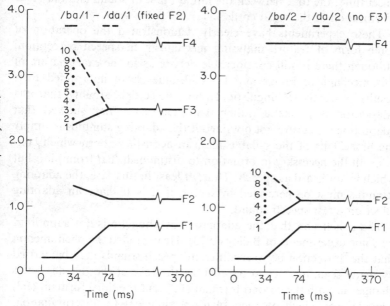

Figure 7.1 Schematic spectrograms of the stimulus sets used by Bailey (1973). In the left-hand half of the figure F2 is fixed and F3 varies. In the right-hand half F2 varies and F3 is absent. In both cases the variation is sufficient to produce a clear perception of /ba/ at one end of the range and /da/ at the other. From Bailey (1973), by permission of the author.

speech sounds (see Chapter 6). Bailey (1973) generated a series of synthetic speech stimuli which were identical except for the first 40 ms. The frequencies of the second and third formants were changed during this initial period, so as to produce a /ba/ sound at one end of the series and a /da/ sound at the other (see Figure 7.1). As we have noted previously, in identifying stimuli from such a series the listeners' responses do not change gradually with changes in the physical stimulus, but change abruptly at some point in the range. Bailey chose an adapting stimulus from one end or the other of the series and presented it to the subject 40 times. He then presented test stimuli chosen to lie around the point on the continuum where the identification normally switches from one syllable to the other. He found that after adaptation to /ba/ an intermediate stimulus was more likely to be perceived as /da/, and vice versa. Other workers have demonstrated similar effects for physical variables such as voice onset time: the time between the initial burst of sound and the onset of vibration of the vocal cords.

These experiments have clearly demonstrated the operation of some form of feature-analysing mechanism in speech perception, although there is still considerable debate as to the exact nature of this mechanism. Eimas and his colleagues have interpreted their results in terms of linguistic feature detectors, arguing that the adaptation is phonetic rather than auditory. They showed that adaptation effects are not obtained if the adapting stimulus is simply the first 50 ms of the syllable /da/, an acoustic pattern which contains all the necessary information to distinguish /ba/ from /da/, but which is not heard as speech. Thus, at least in this case, the adapting stimulus must be perceived in speech if it is to have an adapting effect on a test speech sound.

The conclusion that the adaptation is phonetic is not supported by some experiments of Bailey (1973). He exploited the phenomenon that the distinction between different speech sounds may be carried by many separate cues in parallel. In the case of the /ba–da/ series changes in both the second formant (F2) and the third formant (F3) provide cues which on their own are sufficient for discrimination. Bailey constructed two synthetic /ba–da/ series, one with a fixed F2 and all cues in F3, the other with no F3 and all cues in F2. He found cross-adaptation from the F2 cues series to the fixed F2, but none from the F3 cues series to no F3. On the basis of this experiment, and an additional experiment using a fixed third formant, Bailey concluded: 'When the cues in the adapter and test syllables are carried by different formants, and are hence spectrally well-separated, very little effect of adaptation is observed. This implies that the cues used here to convey the place distinction in these initial consonants are *independently* extracted, rather than being processed as a combined spectral pattern by a higher-level linguistic feature detector.'

Clearly, the issue of auditory versus phonetic detectors is not yet resolved, and it may well be that both types of detectors exist. If phonetic detectors do indeed exist, then this would provide good evidence that the analysis of speech into phonemes is reasonable from a perceptual point of view, but proof of the existence of such detectors would not help us to understand the mechanism by which the complex and variable acoustic cues of speech are decoded into phonemic units. Many curious features of the adaptation process remain to be explained. For example, Bailey (1974) has shown that the adaptation effect is well developed after only eight adapter repetitions, equivalent to about four seconds' exposure to the repeated speech sound. If the effect were the result of fatiguing a particular group of neurones, one would expect a longer build-up than this. Cooper (1974) has shown that adaptation to a particular speech sound may not only affect perceptual boundaries, but also produce correlated shifts in the production of speech sounds. This may indicate a link between the perception and production of speech, as is hypothesised in the motor theory of speech perception (Chapter 6). Research on contingent after-effects in vision has shown that the effects are in many ways more like conditioning than sensory adaptation, and this may well be the case for auditory feature detectors. Thus while these effects are fascinating, and possibly of considerable importance, their exact significance must remain in some doubt.

7.3 PSYCHOACOUSTIC CONSIDERATIONS IN CHOOSING YOUR HI-FI

The last few years have seen a considerable expansion in the sale of sound-reproducing equipment, while at the same time manufacturers have been competing with one another in their efforts to produce 'better' amplifiers, loudspeakers, and so on. Unfortunately, the criterion for 'better' has not usually been clearly defined, and in most cases there has been little effort to investigate the extent to which improvements in technical specification actually produce *audible* improvements. There is, of course, the problem of defining the objectives of high-fidelity reproduction. One aim which has often been put forward is that the sound reproduced in the listening room should be the same for the listener as if he had actually had a good seat at a concert. In most practical situations this aim is unrealistic. Firstly, the echoes and reverberations in a concert hall contribute to the listening experience in a way which cannot be accurately simulated in a normal listening room (although reasonable approximations may be possible using multichannel reproduction). It is only in an anechoic chamber that it is feasible to recreate exactly the sound field that a listener would experience at a live concert (see Section 7.5). Secondly, the peak sound levels occurring at a concert may be high compared with the levels which are practicable or even tolerable in a domestic situation.

In practice recorded sounds may actually be 'better' than sounds heard at a live performance, for a number of reasons. Recording engineers typically use a large number of microphones and a tape recorder with many independent (but synchronised) channels. The engineer is able to position each microphone so as to capture the sound of a particular instrument or group of instruments, and several different types of microphones may be used in order to optimise the recording for each instrument. Sometimes four or five microphones are used to record the drums alone. The final published recording is obtained by 'mixing down' from, say, 24 channels to 2 (for stereo) or 4 (for quadraphonic reproduction). At the stage of mixing down, the engineer and the producer have the option of manipulating the recorded signals in many ways so as to achieve the desired sound quality. For example, the sound spectrum in any of the channels may be altered by banks of filters, so as to produce subtle alterations in timbre or to compensate for the acoustics of the recording room. Cymbals may be made 'crisper', bass notes 'deeper', voices more or less 'breathy', and so on. Reverberation may be added, in controlled amounts and with controlled characteristics, and the impression of the location of different instruments may be controlled by manipulating the amount of sound from each channel which is fed to each of the final channels. In addition, several different recordings of a given piece of music may be taken, and the best sections from each recording spliced together, to give a final performance which is as nearly perfect as possible; even single notes may be spliced in if a musician makes a mistake.

It is generally acknowledged that modern recorded music, reproduced on high-quality equipment, does have advantages over live music in terms of clarity and the definition of individual instruments. Further, many pieces of recorded music could not be produced at a live performance, since they rely on techniques of superimposition of separate recordings and on electronic manipulations which can only be performed in a recording studio. It makes sense, then, to define the object of high-fidelity as the reproduction of sounds corresponding as closely as possible to the intention of the record producer. Thus the emphasis is on accuracy or fidelity of reproduction.

Any high-fidelity reproduction system contains several different components, each of which may alter or distort signals in various ways. The most common system probably involves a record-player (pick-up, arm and turntable), an amplifier and a set of loudspeakers (usually two). Each of these will distort the signal in some way, and for any particular type of distortion the performance of the chain as a whole will be determined by the performance of its weakest link. It is usually true that much more distortion arises in the transducers of the system (the pick-up and the loudspeakers) than in the amplifier; even a cheap amplifier will perform far better than any loudspeaker. Thus audible improvements in a system are much more likely to result from changes in loudspeakers than they are from changes in amplifiers. In the following paragraphs we shall consider in turn each of the major components in a sound-reproducing system, emphasising those aspects of performance which are likely to be most important in how the system *sounds*.

As was mentioned above, the basic performance of even a moderately priced amplifier is likely to be so good that improvements in technical specification would make little audible difference. Nevertheless, some aspects of performance are worth considering. The necessary power output of an amplifier can only be determined in relation to the loudspeakers with which it will be used. Loudspeakers vary considerably in the efficiency with which they convert electrical energy into sound energy; horn loudspeakers may have efficiencies of 30 per cent or more, while 'acoustic suspension' loudspeakers may convert less than 1 per cent of the electrical energy into sound. Thus it is nonsense to say, as one manufacturer has done, that an amplifier produces 'forty-four watts of pure sound'. In fact, even one acoustic watt, in a normal-sized room, would correspond to an extremely loud sound. There are many loudspeakers available which produce high sound levels (in excess of 90 dB SPL) with quite moderate electrical inputs, say 1 W. In other words, given loudspeakers of reasonable efficiency, it is quite unnecessary to spend a lot of money on a high-power amplifier. Additionally, it is worth remembering that a doubling of power (which might mean a doubling in price) produces only a 3 dB change in sound level, which is only just noticeable. On the whole, it is better to buy efficient loudspeakers and an amplifier of moderate power than to buy inefficient loudspeakers and to compensate with a high-power amplifier. Unfortunately, manufacturers have not yet standardised their methods of specifying loudspeaker efficiencies, but the most common way is in terms of the electrical input (in watts) required to produce a sound level of 90 dB SPL at a distance of 1 m from the loudspeaker. Sometimes the level specified is 96 dB SPL, in which case the power required will be four times that needed to produce a level of 90 dB SPL.

One aspect of amplifier performance which is commonly quoted is frequency response. This is measured by using as input to the amplifier a sinewave of constant amplitude but variable frequency. Ideally the output of the amplifier should not vary as a function of frequency, so that all frequencies are amplified to an equal extent. In practice there will be a limit to the range of frequencies which the amplifier will reproduce, and the frequencies at which the output of the amplifier has fallen to one-half power (the 3 dB points) are used to define this range. Modern amplifiers easily out-perform loudspeakers in this respect, and most cover the entire audible range of frequencies (say 20–20 000 Hz) without appreciable fluctuations in output. Some manufacturers have gone to extremes in this respect, presumably to impress unsuspecting customers, and quote frequency responses such as 5–100 000 Hz. It is quite unnecessary, and indeed undesirable, for an amplifier to cover such a wide frequency range. Very-low-frequency components produced by record warps may be of high amplitude, and may overload the amplifier if they are reproduced at full power. In addition, such components can produce very large excursions of loudspeaker cones, which may easily damage them. Frequency components between 20 and 100 kHz will not be audible, but if amplified they may contribute to audible distortion and may present quite a high-power input to the high-frequency unit (tweeter) of a loudspeaker system. Thus the power capacity of both the amplifier and tweeter in reproducing audible frequencies will be limited by the extent to which that power is being wasted in reproducing inaudible high frequencies. In conclusion, the frequency response of an amplifier is rarely a limiting factor in performance, but beware of amplifiers which have frequency responses extending very far beyond the audible range.

Most amplifiers distort signals to some extent. Usually the distortion is specified in terms of the extent to which frequency components are present at the output which were not present at the input of the amplifier. Unfortunately, distortion is not usually specified in a way which allows an easy estimate of its audibility. The most common method is to specify harmonic distortion. A pure tone of a particular frequency is used as input to the amplifier. If the amplifier distorts the signal, the output will not be exactly sinusoidal, but will be a periodic waveform of the same repetition rate as the input. This periodic waveform can be expressed as a fundamental component (of frequency equal to that of the input sinusoid) and a series of harmonics. The total amplitude of the second and higher harmonics, expressed as a percentage of the amplitude of the fundamental, is called the harmonic distortion, and its value may vary from 0.05 per cent or less for a high-quality amplifier to 3 per cent for a moderately priced amplifier. The *audibility* of harmonic distortion is not predictable from this simple percentage, because audibility depends upon the distribution of energy among the different harmonics. If the energy of the distortion products is mainly in the second and third harmonics, then these harmonics will be masked to some extent by the fundamental, and if the signal is a piece of music, they will in any case be masked by the harmonics which are normally present in the input signal. If, on the other hand, the distortion produces high harmonics, then these will be much more easily audible, and subjectively more objectionable. It is not usually possible to determine from the manufacturer's specification what form the harmonic distortion takes, but test reports often mention whether cross-over distortion is present. Cross-over distortion is manifested by 'kinks' in the output waveform where it changes from positive to negative voltage, or vice versa. It is common in transistor amplifiers but very rare in valve amplifiers. The distortion products produced by this distortion are mainly high harmonics, and so this type of distortion may be detected even at levels as low as 0.1 per cent. In an amplifier in which cross-over distortion is absent levels of harmonic distortion of 2–3 per cent would not normally be noticed.

A different way of measuring distortion is to apply two tones of differing frequency to the amplifier input and to measure the levels of other frequencies at the output of the amplifier. Again the levels of the distortion products are usually expressed as a percentage of the level of the primary tones. Each tone will, of course, produce its own harmonic distortion products, but, in addition, there will be frequency components produced by the non-linear interaction of the two tones. If the frequencies of the two input tones are f_1 and f_2, then 'combination' products will be produced with frequencies such as f_1-f_2, f_1+f_2, $2f_1-f_2$, $2f_1+f_2$. This type of distortion is called intermodulation distortion. Once again, it is difficult to predict the audibility of a given percentage of intermodulation distortion in a normal listening situation, since the figures quoted by a manufacturer depend upon the exact frequencies and relative levels of the tones chosen for the test. In general, intermodulation distortion is more easily audible than harmonic distortion, but levels of less than 0.5 per cent are unlikely to be detected.

Studies of the audibility of distortion in recorded music have given widely differing results, with some authors claiming that harmonic distortion of about 5 per cent is not detectable (Jacobs and Wittman, 1964). Unfortunately, the *type* of distortion has not normally been specified in these experiments, so that no generalisations can be made. One fairly consistent finding has emerged, however; the wider the range of audible frequencies produced by the equipment, the lower is the level of distortion which can be detected or tolerated. Thus if very good loudspeakers with a wide frequency range are used, the level of distortion in the amplifier must be lower than if loudspeakers with a limited frequency range are used.

In summary, with loudspeakers of moderate quality there is no point in spending a lot of money on an amplifier in order to achieve levels of harmonic or intermodulation distortion less than about 0.5 per cent. However, this only applies if cross-over distortion is at very low levels. If very-high-quality loudspeakers are used, then it may be worth considering an amplifier with slightly lower distortion levels. In practice most listeners would not notice 3 per cent harmonic distortion, provided that the distortion was concentrated in the lower harmonics.

One other aspect of amplifier performance is worth a brief mention. All amplifiers add a certain amount of undesired noise to the signal. This noise usually takes the form of a low-frequency hum (related to the frequency of the alternating current supply) and a high-frequency hiss. The performance of an amplifier in this respect is usually specified as the ratio of the output power with a relatively high level input signal to the output power due to hum and noise alone. The ratio is normally expressed in decibels, a typical figure being 60 dB. Of course, at a given setting of the amplifier volume control the noise level is constant, but the signal level may vary considerably. Thus, when the signal is at a low level, the signal-to-noise ratio may be much less than 60 dB. The range of levels over which the signal may vary is called the dynamic range, and at a live music performance this range may be considerable (60 dB or more). If such a range occurred in recorded music, then at times the noise level would equal that of the signal and the noise would be very obtrusive. Thus the dynamic range of recorded music is almost always 'compressed' to about 30 dB. This allows satisfactory performance from amplifiers and associated equipment with relatively modest signal-to-noise ratios, and in practice a signal-to-noise ratio of 60 dB or greater is satisfactory in most domestic situations.

Consider now the characteristics of loudspeakers. The efficiency aspect has already been mentioned, and we shall not discuss it further. Just as was the case for an amplifier, the ideal loudspeaker would have a uniform or flat frequency response over the entire audible range; a constant electrical input would lead to a constant sound output, regardless of the frequency of the applied voltage. The degree to which the response of the loudspeaker differs from this ideal can be specified by using the output in response to a given mid-frequency (often 1 kHz) as a reference level. The output at other frequencies can then be specified in relation to this level, and the overall response can be specified in terms of the range of frequencies over which the variations in output level fall within certain limits. Thus the frequency response for a good loudspeaker might be stated as 50–15 000 Hz $\pm$ 5 dB. This would mean that the sound level did not vary over more than a 10 dB range for any frequency from 50 Hz to 15 000 Hz. Notice that in this respect even a good loudspeaker will be much worse than an amplifier, which might have a frequency response of 20–20 000 Hz $\pm$ 1 dB. Many loudspeakers are so bad that the manufacturers do not specify decibel limits in quoting a 'frequency range' for their loudspeakers. *A frequency response without decibel limits is meaningless.* In practice it is only in recent years, with improvements in loudspeaker design, that manufacturers of the better loudspeakers have felt able to quote accurately specified frequency responses, and this is still not common practice for medium- and low-priced loudspeakers.

The frequency response of a loudspeaker is normally measured in an anechoic chamber, so that there is no reflected sound from walls, ceiling and floor which could affect the results. In domestic situations reflected sound will always be present and will influence the overall sound to some extent. High frequencies are usually absorbed more than low frequencies, so that the effective level of the low frequencies is boosted, and this partially compensates for the falling frequency response which is found at low frequencies in most loudspeakers. A second but less desirable effect of reflected sound is that resonances may be set up at particular frequencies, so that when a piece of music is reproduced, those frequencies are more prominent, giving the music an unpleasant 'coloured' sound. The frequencies of the resonances depend upon the dimensions of the listening room; the larger the room the lower will be the frequencies of the resonances. In general, three major resonances will be produced, corresponding to the length, width and height of the room. Ideally none of these dimensions should coincide, otherwise a particularly strong resonance may be produced. The resonances may be 'broken up' by large pieces of furniture, so that their effect is reduced. Thus it is desirable that the listening room should not be too sparsely furnished, but should contain settees, armchairs, and so on.

Given that room acoustics are bound to have an influence on the 'effective' frequency response of a loudspeaker, one might think that the response of a loudspeaker measured in an anechoic chamber is not particularly relevant to how the loudspeaker will sound. This is not in fact the case, because peaks and dips in the 'anechoic' frequency response will combine with peaks and dips produced by room resonances to produce an overall response which is more irregular than either alone. To minimise this irregularity the 'anechoic' frequency response should be as flat as possible. In addition, listeners appear to compensate for the characteristics of a room in judging the nature of a sound source. This is shown by the everyday experience that the quality of the voice of a familiar person does not change markedly with changes in the room in which the person is heard. The effect is an example of perceptual constancy; the properties of an object (in this case a voice) as perceived by an observer vary little with quite large changes in the conditions of observation. It may be that something analogous to the precedence effect (Section 5.5) operates in judgements of sound quality as well as in the localisation of sound. If this were the case, then the perceived quality of a sound would be determined by that part of the sound that reached the ears first, as direct sound from the loudspeaker rather than reflected sound. Thus changes in signals produced by loudspeaker imperfections would be noticed much more than changes produced by room reflections. This is not to deny that room acoustics have an effect, but their effect is less noticeable than might be predicted from physical measurements. As far as loudspeakers are concerned, a frequency response of 50–15 000 Hz ± 3 dB would be exceptionally good, and provided that other aspects of the performance were also good, a loudspeaker with this response would add little of its own quality to the reproduced sound; it would be an accurate transducer.

One aspect of loudspeaker performance which has been largely neglected until recently is the phase response. In order for a waveform to be reproduced accurately not only should all the frequency components be reproduced at the correct relative amplitudes, but also the relative phases of the components should be preserved. This is equivalent to saying that at the listener's ear the time delay of all frequency components should be equal. Changes in the relative phases of the components can produce marked changes in a waveform. Loudspeaker manufacturers have not paid much attention to this, because it has generally been assumed that the ear is insensitive to changes in relative phase. The statement that the ear is phase-deaf is often ascribed to Helmholtz (1863), who experimented with harmonic complex tones containing eight successive harmonics, including the fundamental. In fact, Helmholtz did not exclude the possibility that phase changes were detectable for high harmonics, beyond the sixth to eighth, and more recent work has shown that phase changes produce both changes in timbre (Plomp and Steeneken, 1969) and changes in the clarity of pitch (Bilsen, 1973). The effects for steady tones are, however, rather small. This is not particularly surprising, since, for steady sounds, room reflections will produce marked alternations in the relative phases of components, and we have already seen that room acoustics have relatively little effect on the perceived quality of reproduced sounds. The situation is rather different for transient or short-duration sounds, which are, of course, common in music. The results of a number of experiments have indicated that we can discriminate between sounds differing only in the relative phases of the components (and not in component amplitude), even when those sounds have durations as small as 2–3 ms (Patterson and Green, 1970). When such sounds are reproduced by loudspeakers, any given sound will be completed before any reflected sounds (echoes) reach the ears, provided that the head of the listener is more than 2–3 ft (60–90 cm) from any room surface. Thus room reflections will have little effect on our ability to discriminate between short-duration sounds differing in the relative phases of the components. This has been confirmed by Hansen and Madsen (1974).

What these results mean is that the phase response of a loudspeaker is quite important in determining the subjective quality of the reproduced sound. Changes in the relative phases of components are much more noticeable when those components are close together in frequency than when they are widely separated, so that phase changes which occur abruptly as a function of frequency will have a larger subjective effect than phase changes which occur gradually over a wide frequency range. Unfortunately, the former is the more common situation. Most modern 'high-fidelity' loudspeakers contain two or more transducers to deal with different parts of the frequency range. A 'woofer' is used for low frequencies and a 'tweeter' for high. The electronic input to the loudspeaker is split into high- and low-frequency bands by electronic filters known as cross-over networks, and the transition frequency between a high and a low band is known as the cross-over frequency. It is in the region of the cross-over frequency that rapid phase changes occur, and thus the cross-over network is a source of phase distortion. In addition, certain cabinet designs, such as the vented enclosure or reflex cabinet, introduced marked phase changes in particular frequency regions. It is noteworthy that loudspeakers such as the Quad electrostatic, which use a completely different design avoiding cross-over networks and their consequent phase distortion, are judged to reproduce sounds with greater clarity and realism than most conventional loudspeakers. This is true even of loudspeakers which have more uniform frequency responses than that of the Quad. It seems likely that the differences in phase response play a major role in this subjective evaluation. Recently some manufacturers of conventional loudspeakers have modified their designs so as to produce a much more uniform phase response, and they claim that listeners report a marked preference for these modified loudspeakers. It is to be hoped that in the future manufacturers will pay more attention to the phase response of loudspeakers, and that the aspects of phase response which are subjectively important will become more clearly defined.

A property of loudspeakers which is connected to the phase response is the transient response, which refers to the ability of a loudspeaker to reproduce rapidly changing or short-duration sounds. In theory a loudspeaker with a perfect frequency and phase response would also have a perfect transient response, but since the former are never perfect, some alteration of the temporal characteristics of sounds always occurs. Transient response is often measured with short tone bursts, with a rectangular envelope, which are gated on and off at zero-crossings so as to contain a whole number of periods. Most loudspeakers will not reproduce such a waveform exactly, one common effect being that the abrupt cessation of a tone burst is transformed into an oscillation decaying to zero over several periods. This is known as ringing, and its effect is to lengthen the apparent duration of short sounds and to 'blur' the overall sound quality. Thus excessive ringing in a loudspeaker is undesirable, producing a loss of clarity and definition. It is worth noting that most amplifiers have flat frequency and phase responses with the tone controls in the 'flat' or '12 o'clock' position. If the low frequencies are boosted using the bass control, so as to compensate for a poor low-frequency response in a loudspeaker, then the phase response is markedly altered. If a large boost is required, then quite severe ringing may occur at low frequencies, so that the sound becomes 'boomy'. This again results in a loss of definition, so that it becomes difficult to tell a bowed string from a plucked string. Similar considerations apply to the use of treble controls or high-frequency filters. Thus, while amplifier tone controls can be used to compensate for defects in loudspeaker performance, the corrections if excessive are accompanied by undesirable changes in phase and transient responses. If possible, it is better to use good loudspeakers so that the amplifier can be operated with the controls close to the 'flat' position.

The frequency response of a loudspeaker is usually measured with a microphone directly in front of the loudspeaker, a position known as 'on axis'. If the microphone is placed 'off axis', at some angle to the loudspeaker but at the same distance from it, the measured output will generally fall. This is because the sound is 'beamed' forward by the loudspeaker, rather than being propagated equally in all directions. This beaming is generally much more marked at high frequencies than at low, since it depends upon the wavelength of the sound in relation to the size of the transducer. A very narrow beam of sound at any given frequency is undesirable, since the character of the reproduced sound would be strongly influenced by small changes in the listening position, but the optimum angle of dispersion has not yet been determined, or even investigated in a systematic way. Some manufacturers have gone to extremes in this respect, creating 'omnidirectional' loudspeakers, which radiate sounds equally in all directions for all frequencies. With such loudspeakers the perceived sound quality is relatively independent of listening position, but at the same time certain undesirable effects occur. At the listener's ear the ratio of reflected sounds from walls and ceilings to direct sound will be much greater than for conventional loudspeakers. This makes sound localisation very difficult, since the precedence effect (Section 5.5) may break down when this ratio is too great. In addition, the changes in phase and frequency response produced by room reflections will be subjectively more noticeable, because of the increased proportion of reflected sounds reaching the listener. One further disadvantage occurs when, as is commonly the case, the omnidirectional sound pattern at high frequencies is achieved by using two or more tweeters, each pointing in a different direction. Since the listener will rarely be equally distant from all of the tweeters, their outputs will not arrive in synchrony, but will be staggered in time. A time delay between two sounds is equivalent to a phase shift, but the size of the phase shift will vary with frequency. For some frequencies the phase shift will be close to a whole number of cycles, so that the sound is reinforced, while at other frequencies the phase shift may result in a partial cancellation of the sound. The result is a rippled spectrum, showing a series of maxima and minima as a function of frequency (a similar effect gives rise to the reflection tone which was described in Section 5.13). This gives the sound a marked 'coloration'.

On the whole, most listeners seem to prefer a directional characteristic in which some beaming occurs but where the response is reasonably uniform for an angle of about 45 degrees on either side of the axis. However, individuals may vary considerably in their preferences, so that it is not possible to define a single optimum response. Clearly, this is an area where further research would be very useful.

We have dwelt at some length on the characteristics of loudspeakers, since loudspeakers are usually the 'weakest link' in a sound-reproducing chain, and so they will have the largest effect on how the system will sound. However, the signal source at the start of the chain (e.g. record-player or tape-recorder) may also have a significant effect on the overall sound. Many of the characteristics of pick-ups or cartridges in record-players are defined in a similar way to those of loudspeakers, except that the input signal is a mechanical movement imposed by a record groove and the output is an electrical signal. Thus the same criteria as were used in evaluating loudspeakers can be applied to the evaluation of pick-ups. In general, top-class pick-ups are capable of excellent performance, superior to that of most loudspeakers, in terms of frequency response, transient response and phase response, but this is not always true of cheaper models. However, even high-quality pick-ups produce non-negligible amounts of harmonic and intermodulation distortion, the latter being typically around 2 to 5 per cent. The level of intermodulation distortion may well contribute significantly to the overall sound quality of a pick-up, high levels of distortion being accompanied by a loss of clarity and by a loss of the definition of individual instruments.

Several important aspects of performance are unique to pick-ups. One of these, called tracking, refers to the ability of the stylus to maintain contact with the record grooves in highly modulated (i.e. high-amplitude) passages of the record. In modern recordings the stylus may be subject to accelerations 1000 times the acceleration due to gravity (g), so that it is something of a miracle that good groove contact can be maintained with downward forces on the stylus of one gram or less. When groove contact is partially lost, a condition known as mistracking, the sound may become fuzzy or distorted, or severe crackling may occur. The cure is usually to *increase* the playing weight, provided that it is within the range specified by the manufacturer. Pick-ups vary considerably in their tracking ability, and few manufacturers (with one notable exception) give accurate specifications of this factor; the best that the prospective buyer can do is to rely on test reports. It is worth noting that the tracking ability of a pick-up will only be fully realised if it is used with an arm of appropriate quality. A high-quality pick-up, tracking at one gram or less, requires an arm with very low pivot friction and very low mass.

When stereophonic, or two-channel, reproduction is required, the pick-up must be capable of providing two sets of electrical signals, each one derived from the movement of just one wall of the groove. Two factors are of relevance here: the channel separation and the channel balance. Channel separation is usually measured using a signal recorded so that ideally it would be reproduced in one channel only. The ratio of the output in the desired channel to that in the unwanted channel, expressed in decibels, gives a measure of the extent to which the pick-up can separate the two channels. A figure of 15–20 dB is generally considered adequate, and many pick-ups can easily exceed this. It is important, however, that the separation be maintained over a wide frequency range. Channel balance is measured by recording signals which should be reproduced with equal amplitude on both channels. The ratio of the output levels of the two channels, expressed in decibels, is used as the measure of balance. A difference in level in the two channels which is independent of signal frequency is not important, since it can be corrected using the balance control on the amplifier. However, a difference in level which varies as a function of frequency is more serious. The subjective location of any given instrument in a stereo recording is determined by the relative levels at which the instrument is reproduced by the two loudspeakers. A sound produced equally by the two loudspeakers, and heard by a listener equally distant from them, will be located mid-way between the two loudspeakers. If the sound coming from the left-hand loudspeaker is slightly higher in level than that from the right, then the sound image will be displaced slightly to the left. If the sound from the left-hand loudspeaker is 10–15 dB higher in level than that from the right, the sound will be located entirely at the left-hand loudspeaker. Clearly, then, channel balance is important in determining the subjective location of individual instruments. If the balance varies as a function of frequency, then different frequency components produced by the same instrument will be subjectively located in different places. Thus there will not be a well-defined 'stereo image'. Instead the 'image' corresponding to any given instrument will be diffuse, and the separation of individual instruments will be reduced. Similar considerations apply to the two loudspeakers of a stereo pair; these should be matched as closely as possible in terms of frequency and phase response, otherwise the 'stereo image' will suffer.

Finally, we will consider briefly the characteristics of turntables. These may affect sound quality in two ways. Firstly, mechanical vibrations in the turntable itself may be detected by the pick-up and reproduced as a rumbling sound. Secondly, the fluctuations in the speed of the turntable produce corresponding fluctuations in the frequencies of the reproduced sounds. Slow fluctuations, called wow, produce pitch changes which are particularly noticeable on steady piano tones, while rapid fluctuations, called flutter, give the sound a 'rough' quality. Rumble is usually specified by measuring its level in relation to a tone recorded at a particular reference level, most often a 1 kHz pure tone at a groove velocity (in the lateral direction) of 10 cm/s. A good figure for a high-quality turntable would be −45 dB. Although this does not look very good as a noise-to-signal ratio, it should be remembered that rumble is composed mainly of very-low-frequency components (usually below 100 Hz), and the ear is not very sensitive to these low frequencies (see Figure 2.1). Some manufacturers have tried to take this into account by using a weighting characteristic which reduces the contribution of very low frequencies. The principle is similar to that used in the loudness level meters which were described in Section 2.3. This results in rumble-to-signal ratios which look very much more favourable; figures of -65 to -70 dB are not unusual. As yet there has been no systematic study to determine whether the weighted or the unweighted measure gives a closer correlation with the degree of annoyance produced by the rumble. The extent to which rumble is audible will, of course, depend on the ability of the loudspeakers to reproduce low frequencies. Consequently, high-quality loudspeakers, with a good low-frequency response, should be accompanied by a turntable with minimal rumble. Wow and flutter are not normally noticeable unless their level exceeds about 0.3 per cent, although somewhat lower levels of wow may just be detectable in sustained tones. Levels of wow and flutter less than 0.1 per cent would certainly not be detectable, and such levels are relatively common in modern turntables.

In summary, in the selection of components for a high-fidelity system it is important that no component be selected in isolation. Rather each component must be chosen so as to be compatible in quality with the other components. If funds are limited, then the best performance will be obtained by buying efficient loudspeakers, which will produce sufficiently high sound levels using an amplifier of moderate power. However, many of the highest-quality loudspeakers are relatively inefficient, and if such loudspeakers are to be used, a high-power amplifier may be necessary. An inefficient loudspeaker may require 100 times the power of an efficient loudspeaker to produce the same sound level, so if a 1 W amplifier were sufficient for the former, a 100 W amplifier would be needed for the latter. The record-playing equipment (turntable, arm and pick-up) should be chosen after the loudspeakers. The better the quality of the loudspeakers, the more likely they will be to show up faults in the record player. The loudspeakers and pick-up are by far the most critical components of a Hi-Fi system, but many of the factors which influence sound quality are not specified by manufacturers, or are specified in ways which are not easily related to subjective impressions. In addition, the importance of such factors as phase response and directional characteristics has not yet been established. Thus it is difficult to determine from manufacturers' specifications how good a given pick-up or loudspeaker will sound. If possible, the best way to choose these components is by listening to them, preferably using a familiar well-recorded record, and preferably in one's own home.

To conclude this section we shall briefly discuss multichannel sound reproduction. Stereophonic or two-channel reproduction, as

17-2

was mentioned above, creates the impression of instruments located in different positions in space by varying the relative levels of different instruments in the two channels. For sounds which are emitted solely from one or the other loudspeaker there is no problem in subjectively locating the sound source, but for sounds which are intended to be heard as coming from between the two loudspeakers there is sometimes a problem. The sounds reaching the listeners' ears are, in fact, quite different from those which would have been produced by a real sound source lying between the loudspeakers, and for many listeners the reproduced sound of a given instrument does not occupy any single position in space, but is broadened, or spread out, between the two loudspeakers. Thus stereophonic reproduction is limited both in its ability to create a precise impression of the location of different instruments and by the fact that the range of possible subjective locations is limited to a horizontal arc between (and sometimes slightly beyond) the two loudspeakers. However, for most listeners the main benefit of stereophonic reproduction over monophonic (single-channel) reproduction is not connected with localisation *per se*, but rather with improved clarity and definition, so that individual instruments can be heard more precisely. This effect is probably related to the BMLD phenomenon, which was discussed in Sections 5.8–5.10.

In recent years various forms of multichannel reproduction have been introduced, the most common approach being to use four channels, but there is no clear consensus of opinion as to the object of such systems, or their expected advantages. It is worthwhile to distinguish between the number of separate channels of auditory information and the number of loudspeakers over which the sounds are reproduced. An ordinary stereo record can carry two effectively independent sets of auditory information, but these two sets can be processed and replayed via any number of loudspeakers. For example, the two conventional loudspeakers can be retained, but a third loudspeaker, receiving inputs equally from the two channels, can be placed between them. Many of the 'four-channel' systems currently in use, the so-called matrix systems, actually use only two independent sets of information, the outputs to the four loudspeakers being derived from these two channels. Thus conventional stereo records, or two-channel tape-recorders, can be used, but the signals emitted by the four loudspeakers are not independent of one another. This is not necessarily a disadvantage. Other four-channel systems, those called discrete, do actually use four independent sets of information, but in order to do so they require either a four-channel tape-recorder or a special kind of record in which a high-frequency tone is recorded and used to decode the two stereo channels into four channels.

In most of the four-channel systems which are currently available 'quadraphonic' reproduction is really just an extension of stereophonic reproduction. The direction of sound sources is encoded by pairwise blending between loudspeakers associated with adjacent corner positions. As we saw above, conventional stereo systems are not very good in creating a precise impression of location, and the problems associated with this kind of approach become even more marked for pairs of loudspeakers lying to the side of, or behind, the listener. Thus, although quadraphonic systems can be used to broaden the range of subjective locations associated with the re-produced instruments, the improvement in this respect is severely limited.

A phrase which is often used in conjunction with quadraphonics is 'surround-sound', although, as Fellgett (1974) has pointed out, the two are not identical, and surround-sound can be achieved with fewer than four channels. For Fellgett one of the most important factors in sound reproduction is connected with the reverberation or ambience of the concert hall in which the performance takes place. He points out that each instrument, by virtue of its location, will have associated with it a particular set of echoes. Thus each section of the orchestra is 'labelled with an acoustic ambience characteristic of its place of origin'. This leads Fellgett to conclude that '. . . the highest fidelity in sound reproduction requires that the directionality of sound should mimic both the direct and the reverberant sound of the concert hall. This is not just a matter of a vague splash of delayed echoes, but of a relationship between directionality and time delay which gives specific information; this information is what we shall mean by ambience. Systems capable of reproducing it will be called "ambisonic".'

As was mentioned at the beginning of this section, it is not possible to mimic exactly in a normal room the sound field which a listener would have experienced at a live concert. However, Fellgett has reported that with suitable recording and processing techniques a reasonable approximation can be obtained using a relatively small number of channels and loudspeakers. For a system in which only horizontal direction information is preserved (Fellgett calls this a pantophonic system) two independent channels and four loud-speakers seem to provide a subjectively satisfactory approximation. Unfortunately, there has been no published work in which subjects have judged the merits of this system as compared with other systems under appropriately controlled listening conditions. The ambisonic approach undoubtedly does have something to offer. Gerzon (1971) found that correctly recorded reverberation did aid sound localisation during reproduction, while poor artificial reverberation made the sound image less distinct. However, the technique is limited in the accuracy with which the original sound field can be reproduced. The accuracy is least at high frequencies, where pinnae encoding effects become significant, and this means that the localisation information at high frequencies will conflict to some extent with that at low frequencies. In addition, the acoustics of the listening room will always influence the reproduced sound field in a largely uncontrolled way. Ambisonic recordings are made with a microphone array at some distance from the instruments, usually at a position which would have been occupied by the listener's head. This is necessary for the encoding of the reverberation information. However, this approach is incompatible with the close-microphone techniques which are commonly used in recording studios and which contribute so much to the quality and clarity of modern recordings. Thus the ambience information is gained at the expense of a possible loss of clarity, while at the same time the record-producer has much less flexibility in terms of adjusting the balance of the various instruments and manipulating their sound qualities. The preferences of the listening audience will ultimately determine which approach is the more successful.

One sound-reproduction technique which has been developed in the past few years does appear to be remarkably successful in creating for the listener an impression similar to that which he would have obtained at a live concert. This technique uses a dummy head, whose acoustic properties are designed to mimic those of the human head and pinnae as closely as possible. The recording is made via microphones which are placed in positions corresponding to the eardrums of the dummy head. Thus the sound picked up by the microphones is very close to that which would have been heard by a listener. The recorded sounds are replayed via headphones and the result can be astonishingly realistic. According to Stahl (1975),

'... sound sources are correctly localised outside the head; various distances from a few centimetres to more than 100 m are reproduced precisely; the timbre corresponds to the distance from the sound source; the impression of reverberation is natural; all directions of sound incidence, from the left, right, front, from behind, above and below can be distinguished'. The system, in addition, has the advantage of requiring only two channels, so that existing recording media can be used.

Experimental radio broadcasts of dummy-head recordings, which have been transmitted in West Germany, have generally met with an enthusiastic response from the public, although it is not at the present time clear whether this enthusiasm is partly a response to the novelty of the effects. The system is certainly not without its drawbacks. Not all individuals are satisfied with the accuracy of subjective location produced, although the reasons for this are not entirely clear. One possible factor is that the signals essentially pass through an ear canal twice, which produces changes in phase and frequency response. (This can be corrected using appropriate filters.) A second factor is that pinnae differ slightly from person to person, so that the dummy head will not precisely mimic the head of any given listener. A more serious effect is that the cues to auditory localisation which normally are produced by head movements are completely absent in dummy-head recordings. Indeed, rather than producing additional cues, movements of the listener's head produce changes in the apparent orientation of the orchestra and concert hall, which is a disconcerting effect. It is likely that cues relating to head movements are normally of considerable importance in the location of sounds in the frontal plane, and in distinguishing front from back, and it is noteworthy that in dummy-head recordings the least accurately defined positions tend to be at the front (Gerzon, 1975). Stahl (1975) has suggested that this problem could be at least partially eliminated by monitoring the movements of the subject's head and using these movements to introduce appropriate time and intensity differences between the two ears. This solution would be expensive, and probably impracticable in a domestic situation. One final criticism of the dummy-head technique is similar to the one applied to ambisonics. The clarity and definition which is achieved on modern recordings is made possible by the separate recording of individual instruments or groups of instruments. This method also allows subsequent alterations in musical balance and corrections of the imperfections of individual instruments. A dummy-head recording provides a means of reproducing the total orchestral sound at a particular seat in a particular concert hall, which generally does not allow such clear discrimination of individual instruments and which carries with it any limitations in musical balance and concert hall acoustics. Once again, the preferences of listeners must ultimately be the factor determining the future of these systems.

7.4 APPLICATIONS OF PSYCHOACOUSTIC RESEARCH IN THE ALLEVIATION OF DEAFNESS

Audiology is the science of the evaluation of hearing, particularly in relation to the hearing-impaired. On the basis of an audiological examination, particular types of hearing disorders may be diagnosed and particular types of hearing-aids recommended. Psychoacoustics is the scientific basis of audiology, and most tests in clinical audiology are based on the findings of psychoacoustic research and on changes in psychoacoustic phenomena which may occur in different disorders of the auditory pathways. Some of these have been discussed already in Chapter 2.

The basic difference between audiology and psychoacoustics lies in the methodology employed. A psychoacoustician may have a theoretical interest in quite small and subtle effects, and may be willing to test individual subjects for many hours and/or to average results across a large number of subjects, in order to investigate these effects. The audiologist, on the other hand, requires tests which can be applied quickly and simply to a particular patient, in order to determine the nature of the disorder and localise the site of the auditory lesion. This difference in approach, although it is quite obvious, has nevertheless considerably impeded the interchange of results and ideas between the two disciplines.

There are several areas in which psychoacoustics may be able to make useful contributions in the treatment of the hearing-impaired. One is in the development of new tests which can be used in clinical situations to investigate particular aspects of hearing disorders. The need for such tests is particularly evident in cases of sensori-neural hearing loss, where at the present time there may be problems both in diagnosing the site of the lesion and in predicting the extent of the difficulties which the patient may encounter in everyday life. A related area in which there is scope for considerable improvement is in the choice of a particular hearing-aid for a particular subject. At the present time there is a huge variety of hearing-aids available (the list published by the Royal National Institute for the Deaf in February 1975 contained over 200 different aids), each of which has its own particular characteristics such as high or low gain, wide or narrow frequency response, a frequency response tailored to the subject's audiogram, directional microphones, compression amplification, etc. Unfortunately, there is a paucity of systematic research on which type of aid is best for which type of hearing disorder, and the 'prescription' of a hearing-aid is often made by inspired guesswork rather than on the basis of sound scientific evidence.

In order to evaluate an aid it is essential to maintain contact with the patient, to see that the patient is using the aid in the most appropriate way and to determine whether, in fact, the aid is of real benefit. It is in this area that there is scope for the application of psychoacoustic methods. In order to determine the benefits of any particular aid for a patient, it is necessary to conduct an extensive series of tests using a great variety of materials, and to allow the patient the opportunity of learning to make full use of the acoustic cues provided by the aid. It may be that a series of such studies would allow the formulation of general rules for determining the best type of aid for a particular type of disorder. It is the experience of clinical audiologists that some rules of this type are already known, but that the results of their application are not always predictable. A set of hearing-aids which have very similar specifications on paper may nevertheless perform very differently when fitted to a patient. This provides some justification for trial-and-error methods, but it would clearly be more satisfactory if the reasons for the discrepancies were known. More research is needed into those aspects of hearing-aid performance which are at present poorly specified but which may have important effects on an aid's usefulness to a patient. These include frequency response (which is usually measured via couplers or artificial ears, giving results which are known to be different from those obtained on real ears), harmonic distortion, intermodulation and transient distortion, the effect of different ear-mould fittings, and the effect of different attack and release times in compression hearing-aids. Improvements in the performance of hearing-aids and in their selection for particular patients will only be achieved by isolating those aspects of performance which are most important from the point of view of the patient, and this will require careful psychoacoustic testing.

One relatively new and exciting area of research aims to bring help to those people who are totally deaf through disorders of the sensory organ—the cochlea. The number of people in this category is not clearly known, but may be considerable. In the USA there are 200 000–300 000 people who are so deaf that they cannot hear anything using a conventional hearing-aid. In a large proportion of these the disorder is in the sensory organ rather than in the central nervous system, and the auditory nerve is partially intact (but degenerated to some extent) in the majority of individuals. In such people it is possible to create a sensation of sound by direct electrical stimulation of the auditory nerve. This occurs because of the way in which the auditory nerve is connected to the central nervous system; nerve impulses in the auditory nerve lead to activity in those parts of the brain that are normally concerned with the analysis and perception of sounds, and are interpreted by those parts of the brain as having arisen from acoustic stimulation. Thus, as Merzenich *et al.* (1974) have put it: 'The reasoning behind current efforts to develop acoustic prostheses is that one can generate some facsimile of the normal input that the acoustic nerve receives when stimulated with normal sounds, and thereby generate sensation that constitutes a facsimile of normal sound sensation.'

The extent to which a 'normal sound sensation' can be achieved is still in considerable doubt, and many fundamental questions remain to be answered. However, it has become clear that the problem requires a multidisciplinary approach, with the co-operation of surgeons, neurophysiologists, audiologists, engineers, speech researchers and psychoacousticians. The early work in this field involved the implantation of single bipolar electrodes, which excited simultaneously a large proportion of neurones in the auditory nerve. For surgical reasons it has proved easiest to excite those neurones which would normally respond to high-frequency sounds and would derive their input from the basal part of the cochlea (Simmons, 1966; Merzendich *et al.*, 1973b). Psychoacoustic experiments on patients with these electrodes have revealed that 'sounds' can be heard for a wide range of electrical frequencies of stimulation (25–10 000 Hz), but changes in sensation with changes in rate of stimulation only occur for rates below about 600 Hz. The apparent 'pitch' of electrical stimuli derived by scaling procedures (see Chapter 2) increased regularly with frequency for frequencies up to 500–600 Hz, but then flattened off. Relatively small differences in frequency could be detected. For example, one subject of Merzenich *et al.* (1973b) could detect changes of 2 Hz at 100 Hz, 7 Hz at 200 Hz, 9 Hz at 500 Hz and 60 Hz at 900 Hz. These values are larger than are found in normal subjects, for 'real' sounds, but at low frequencies the discrepancies are not all that large.

The interpretation of these results is somewhat controversial. Clearly, since the same population of neurones is excited by the electrode whatever the rate of stimulation, the changes in sensation with changing frequency must have been coded by changes in the time pattern of neural impulses. Thus these results provide some support for the temporal or periodicity theory of pitch perception which was discussed in Chapter 4. However, the upper frequency limit for which frequency changes could be detected was considerably lower than the limit for which temporal information is available in the normal auditory nerve (4–5 kHz), and the ability to detect changes in frequency was poorer than is found in normal subjects. This has led some workers to suggest that in normal listeners the place cues are the most important and that the use of temporal information is restricted to very low frequencies. It should be remembered, however, that the electrodes in these experiments were stimulating those neurones which normally respond to the high-frequency components of a sound. It may well be the case that the temporal information can only be utilised when it exists in the appropriate neural channels. We know, for example, that residue pitches cannot be heard when all the frequency components in the stimulus lie above 5 kHz (Section 4.3.1). The high-frequency channels involved may be capable of decoding temporal information to some extent, and, indeed, in normal listeners such channels may carry useful information about the envelope periodicity of stimuli (see Sections 4.3.4, 5.3 and 6.4). However, in order to mimic more closely the normal use of temporal information, it may be necessary to stimulate neurones with lower characteristic frequencies.

A second serious problem with this work is that no-one is quite sure what kind of electrical stimulation to use in order to mimic the patterns of neural activity which would be produced by an acoustic stimulus. The two most commonly used types of stimulation have been sinusoidal waves and periodic impulses, but it is clear that neither of these is entirely satisfactory. Unfortunately, the transduction process in the normal ear is not fully understood, so we do not know what the 'normal' input to the auditory nerve is like. More research in this area is clearly needed. At the present time the problem is being tackled by implanting stimulating electrodes in animals and by recording responses in the nervous systems of the animals in response to electrical stimulation. Usually the animals are treated with kanamycin, or some similar drug, which destroys the hair cells of the cochlea. This ensures that neural responses are the results of electrical stimulation and are not mediated by the cochlea. While it has not been possible to define the 'best' method of electrical stimulation, such experiments have provided useful information, both about the effects of stimulating waveform and about the site of stimulation.

The studies on human patients have demonstrated that substantial benefit can be gained by the totally deaf from a single stimulating electrode. The sound sensations, crude though they are, provide valuable contact with the environment and act as warning signals. It is also clear that it will not be possible, using a single electrode, to generate a neural input which would be sufficient for the coding of speech. This is because speech discrimination requires a simultaneous representation of several different frequency components of the stimulus. This can only be achieved by exploiting the place organisation of the auditory nervous system, i.e. by exciting independently several different sets of neurones, each with its own characteristic frequency. Preliminary work on multichannel electrical stimulation has been done, using animal subjects, and the technique does appear to be feasible. Merzenich *et al.* (1974) have developed and tested an electrode suitable for implantation into the scala tympani in man. The scala tympani is one of the fluid-filled chambers of the cochlea, which is relatively easy to approach surgically, and which gives good access to the array of nerve fibres forming the auditory nerve. Michelson *et al.* have pointed out that it might be possible to excite predetermined sectors of the auditory nerve from within the scala tympani if two conditions can be met. These conditions are: (1) the nerve must survive long-term cochlear implantation; (2) the resistance to current flow in the scala tympani must be sufficiently great to restrict stimulation to a reasonably small group of fibres. There has been considerable debate over both of these points, but preliminary results are favourable. The auditory nerve does appear to survive the implantation, for at least several months, and discrete stimulation of groups of fibres within the auditory nerve does appear to be possible.

One problem with the multiple-electrode approach is that the perceptual effects of multiple stimulation are completely unknown and difficult to guess. In the normal listener speech is perceived as a single and complex stream of sound, and not as a series of isolated buzzes, bleeps and hisses. The integration of information from the different frequency components of speech is an essential feature of normal speech perception. We do not know whether such integration will be possible in the patient with an implanted array of electrodes. We saw in Chapter 6 that there is good evidence for a special 'speech mode' of auditory perception, which is triggered by sounds having appropriate characteristics. We do not know whether for the patient with an implanted electrode array the sensations will be too different from those normally associated with speech for the 'speech mode' to be engaged.

The work on electrical stimulation of the auditory nerve is still in its infancy, and many questions remain to be answered. The results of implanting single electrodes have clearly been of use to the patients, providing a valuable link with the outside world, but the sound sensations produced have been crude and comparatively limited. The work using multiple electrode arrays looks more promising, although even with such arrays it will only be possible to simulate very crudely the patterns of neural activity which would occur in the normal ear in response to sound stimuli. The sound sensation is unlikely ever to come close to that of a normal-hearing listener. Most workers in this area would be happy if stimulation with multiple electrodes allowed sufficient information to be transmitted to the auditory nerve for some speech discrimination to be possible. If this aim is to be realised, it will be necessary to carefully investigate the types of training procedures which would best help the patient in learning to use the unfamiliar auditory sensations produced by electrical stimulation. A problem closely coupled to this is that of determining the best way of converting acoustic stimuli into sets of electrical stimuli suitable for driving an array of implanted electrodes. A possible strategy would be to split the acoustic stimulus into several different frequency bands and to feed electrical signals corresponding to the energy in each band separately to different electrodes. Ideally, the characteristic frequency of the small group of neurones excited by any given electrode would be determined previously, so that electrical stimuli derived from acoustic energy in that same frequency region could be delivered to that electrode. Unfortunately, this may not be possible in practice. Most of the information in speech is carried by mid-frequencies, whereas it is easiest to implant electrodes which excite neurones with high characteristic frequencies.

It is possible that some useful insights into the possible effects of the 'mismatching' between acoustic energy and stimulated neurones could be achieved by psychoacoustic tests on normal subjects in which stimuli have been processed so as to mimic, as closely as possible, such mismatching. For example, speech sounds could be processed so that all the frequency components were shifted upwards, and the effects of this on intelligibility could be determined. Given that such processing would certainly have some deleterious effects on intelligibility, it would also be of interest to determine the extent to which subjects can learn to deal with this. Similar tests could be carried out to determine the minimum number of independent 'channels' required for satisfactory speech discrimination. This could be achieved by splitting the speech stimuli into a number of separate frequency bands, each approximately one critical band in width. The minimum number of such channels necessary for satisfactory discrimination could then be determined as a function of their spacing and positioning on the frequency scale. Finally, it would be possible to investigate the combined effects of limiting the number of channels and translating them to a different part of the frequency scale. Such psychoacoustic tests could provide very useful guidelines in determining the optimum spacing and positioning of the electrodes in a multielectrode stimulator, as well as in the design of drivers for converting acoustic signals into sets of electrical signals for delivery to the electrodes. The tests might also be useful in determining appropriate training methods and in indicating the degree of speech intelligibility which can reasonably be expected from an implant with a given number of independent electrodes. It may turn out that quite complicated signal processing will be required in order to realise the full potential of an implanted electrode array, and that the optimum type of processing will differ from patient to patient. If this is the case, then it will be necessary to construct highly versatile driving systems, which can be tailored to individual needs.

It will be many years before the full potential of the cochlear implant is realised, but the first important steps have been taken. We do not know whether such implants will ever allow the deaf to discriminate speech efficiently in everyday conditions, but even if they do not, it is very likely that *some* useful information about speech could be communicated, and this would provide a valuable supplement to other cues such as lip-reading, signing, etc. It is possible that, even with a single stimulating electrode, useful information about the fundamental frequency of a human voice could be communicated. This would allow the deaf person to judge the pitch, and thus the intonation, of the spoken message. In addition, the presence or absence of periodic (i.e. pitch-like) stimulation could be used to signal whether speech sounds were voiced or not. This is a very important distinction for the normal listener, but one which is very difficult to make for the lip-reader. For the profoundly deaf subject the communication of cues relating to intonation and voicing would constitute a major breakthrough.

7.5 THE EVALUATION OF CONCERT HALL ACOUSTICS

This topic is one of great complexity, and it is beyond the scope of this book to cover it in any detail. The interested reader is referred to Beranek (1962) for further details. We shall content ourselves with a brief review of some recent techniques which go a considerable way towards solving the problems inherent in the comparison of concert hall acoustics.

Judgements of the acoustic quality of concert halls, and comparisons between different concert halls, are difficult because of two major factors. Firstly, the perceived quality at a given performance will depend as much on the manner of playing of the musicians and their seating arrangements as on the characteristics of the hall itself. Secondly, long-term acoustical memory is relatively poor, so that many of the subtleties of acoustical quality will not be recalled by the time a listener has travelled from one hall to another. Ultimately the consensus of opinion of a large number of listeners will determine whether a hall is 'good' or 'bad', but it is not easy to determine the crucial features which influence such judgements, or to derive general rules which could be applied in the design of new halls. Indeed, many new halls are simply modelled on other halls which have been judged as good. While this approach does have some validity, it is also very inflexible.

Schroeder, Gottlob and Siebrasse (1974) have developed recording and reproduction techniques which make possible instantaneous comparisons of the acoustic qualities of different halls under realistic free-field conditions on the basis of identical musical source material. The first step is to use as a source material a recording of an orchestra which is played from the stage. This ensures that the musical material is always identical. The orchestra is recorded in an anechoic chamber, so that the acoustics of the recording room are not superimposed on those of the hall being tested. Schroeder *et al.* used a two-channel recording, replayed via two loudspeakers on the stage of the hall, so as to simulate in a crude way the spatial extent of the orchestra. However, there is no reason why the technique should not be extended to multichannel recordings, which would mimic more accurately the sounds radiated by a live orchestra.

The second step is to record the signals using microphones at the 'ear-drums' of a dummy head, as we described in the previous section. Two different positions were used for each hall, both corresponding to places which would normally be occupied by a listener's head. Care was taken to ensure that the acoustic properties of the dummy head, including the ear canal and pinnae, were as accurate as possible.

The third step is to present the dummy-head recordings to listeners for evaluation. One obvious way of doing this is to replay the signals via stereo headphones, but, as we discussed in the previous section, this technique does have its limitations. One problem which Schroeder *et al.* mention is that '. . . listening over earphones does not properly recreate the perceived acoustic "space" or the sense of being surrounded by sound, which is one of the important qualities that we wish to describe in an objective way'. To overcome this problem the recordings were electronically processed so that, when played back over two selected loudspeakers in an anechoic chamber, the recorded signals were recreated at the eardrums of a human listener. Schroeder *et al.* explain the technique as follows: 'The sound radiated from each loudspeaker goes into *both* ears and not just the "near" ear of the listener as would be desired. In other words, there is "cross-talk" from each loudspeaker to the "far" ear. However, by radiating properly mixed and filtered compensation signals from the loudspeakers, the unwanted "cross-talk" can be cancelled out.' The appropriate filter responses in the compensation scheme are computed from measurements obtained by applying short electrical impulses to one of the two loudspeakers and recording the resulting microphone signals from the ears of a dummy head at some distance in front of the loudspeakers. For further details the reader is referred to the original article and to Schroeder and Atal (1963).

The result of this is that, when the original dummy-head recording is replayed, '. . . the signal from the dummy's right ear will go *only* to the listener's right ear and that from the dummy's left ear will go only to the listener's left ear, just as in earphone listening but with the proper free-field coupling of the ear canal and the desired invariance of the perceived acoustical space when the listener's head is rotated around a vertical axis'. Schroeder *et al.* report that for head movements up to about ± 10 degrees the externalised sound image remains stationary with respect to the listening room, and does not turn with the head as in earphone listening.

Using this technique, Schroeder *et al.* asked subjects to indicate preferences for different concert halls presented in pairs. For a given pair the subject was allowed to switch back and forth between recordings made in the two halls as often as he liked. The score for a preferred hall was 1, and for the other − 1. If there was no preference, both halls were given a score of 0. This was repeated for all subjects and all pairs of halls, and the resulting scores were accumulated in a preference matrix indicating how many times each hall was preferred by each listener.

The results were subjected to a factor analysis (Slater, 1960) which yielded the significant factors accounting for the variance in the data. There was one factor of overriding significance, accounting for 50 per cent of the relative variance, which was called the consensus preference factor. All subjects showed positive weights on this factor. What this means is that if a given hall (say X) has a greater value on this factor than another hall (say Y), then hall X is preferred over hall Y by *all* listeners. The other factors isolated by the analysis seem to represent individual-difference preferences. The original recordings were made in unoccupied halls. This has little effect on the acoustics in modern halls, but in older halls with hard wooden seats it can result in excessively long reverberation times. When the analysis was limited to those halls having reverberation times less than 2.2 s, the consensus preference factor became even more important, accounting for 88 per cent of the total variance, while individual preference factors became much less significant.

Schroeder *et al.* also made various physical measurements in the halls, in order to correlate the consensus preference factor with the geometrical and acoustical parameters of the halls. We will not detail all of the measures they considered, but will mention those that appeared to be most significant. For the halls with reverberation times less than 2.2 s. reverberation time was highly correlated with preference. Thus the greater the reverberation time the greater was the consensus. However, for the halls with reverberation times greater than 2 s the reverberation time is slightly negatively correlated with consensus preference, but shows a fairly large correlation with the first individual difference factor. Thus, in this range of reverberation times, some listeners prefer greater reverberation times and others smaller reverberation times.

One factor which showed a strong negative correlation with preference, for halls with both long and short reverberation times, was the interaural coherence. This is a measure of the correlation of the signals at the two ears. Thus listeners prefer halls which produce a low interaural coherence, so that the signals at the two ears are relatively independent of one another. Schroeder *et al.* suggested that 'This effect might be mediated by a more pronounced feeling—of being immersed in the sound—that presumably occurs for less coherent ear signals.' It is possible that the interaural coherence can be manipulated by sound diffusers on the walls and ceiling of the concert hall.

Finally, for the halls with longer reverberation times, which also tended to be the larger halls, the volume of the halls showed a strong negative correlation with consensus preference. Thus, once a hall has reached a certain size, further increases in size result in a worsening of acoustic quality.

The work we have described is very much a beginning in this area, and there are a number of ways in which the techniques could be improved and extended. The number of channels and loudspeakers used in the reproduction of the original sound source on the stage of the concert hall could be increased, a greater variety of musical material could be used, and the dummy head could be positioned so as to sample a greater number of points within each hall. A further possibility, described by Schroeder *et al.*, is to transform all the recordings, using a computer, so that they have the same reverberation time! It is known that reverberation time plays a large part in preference judgements, and when there are large differences in reverberation times, this tends to obscure other factors which might affect preference. By working with the processed recordings, a set of halls with identical reverberation times can be obtained, so that other factors can be more easily isolated.

7.6. GENERAL DISCUSSION AND FUTURE OUTLOOK

The preceding sections have described a few of the ways in which studies of auditory perception have had, or may have in the future, practical applications. There are, of course, many other ways in which sounds may influence our lives. Miller (1974), in a review of the effects of noise on people, described the value of sound in the following way: 'Thus, sound is of great value to man. It warns him of danger and appropriately arouses and activates him. It allows him the immeasurable advantage of speech and language. It can calm, excite, and it can elicit joy or sorrow. The recent discovery that five-day-old infants will work to produce a variety of sounds (Butterfield and Siperstein, 1970) only reinforces the everyday observation that man enjoys hearing and making sounds.'

It may be that future research will pay greater heed to the mood-influencing and aesthetic properties of sound. These properties are not, of course, independent of the purely perceptual aspects of sounds which have been emphasised in this book. In the future composers will no doubt exploit the increasing flexibility in the generation of novel sounds which is provided by modern electronic circuits and computers. This will free them from the limitations of conventional instruments, but will require that they have considerable insight into the perceptual effects of the novel sounds. Psychoacoustics may have a great deal to offer in the development of new forms of music, and in generally increasing our understanding of musical appreciation.

Unfortunately, sound can also have ugly, annoying or unpleasant effects. Miller (1974) has described many of these effects, and we shall content ourselves with a brief summary of his conclusions. Noise of sufficient intensity and duration can permanently damage the inner ear, with resulting permanent hearing losses that can range from slight impairment to nearly total deafness. This was discussed briefly in Section 2.7. There is a clear need for increasing monitoring of public noise exposure and audiometric monitoring of the population at risk. In this way individuals who are particularly susceptible to noise damage could be isolated before the damage becomes severe. There is also a need for education and information to create and enhance public awareness of noise as a hazard to hearing. In addition to actually damaging hearing, noise can have the following undesirable effects: it can interfere with speech communication and the

18-2

perception of other auditory signals; it can disturb sleep; it can be a source of annoyance; it can interfere with the performance of complicated tasks, especially when speech communication or response to auditory signals is demanded; it can reduce the opportunity for privacy; it can adversely influence mood and disturb relaxation. It is to be hoped that an increasing awareness of these effects will lead to improved noise control in the design of buildings, vehicles, machinery and the environment as a whole.

Our knowledge of the processes involved in the perception of sound has advanced considerably since the pioneering work of Helmholtz (1863), yet the scientific study of hearing is still in its infancy. At the physiological level we now know a good deal about the coding of sounds in the auditory nerve, and the cochlear nucleus, but relatively little is known of how that basic neural information is processed at higher levels in the auditory system. At the perceptual level we know a good deal about people's abilities to detect changes in simple stimuli such as pure tones and bands of noise, but we are a long way from understanding how complex auditory patterns such as speech and music are perceived. Unfortunately, the elementary level of our understanding is not accompanied by simplicity in the concepts involved. Many students are deterred by the technical jargon which appears in scientific papers on auditory perception or the neurophysiology or anatomy of the auditory system. For students without a physics background even the nature of auditory stimuli, and their analysis in terms of Fourier components, may present considerable conceptual difficulties. It is my hope that readers who have reached this point in the book by working through the previous chapters will have overcome these initial difficulties, and that some real feeling will have been developed for the fascinating and complex processes that underlie our perception of sound. For those who like to start at the end, let me urge you not to be discouraged. Understanding may seem like a distant light at the end of a long dark tunnel, but the light can be reached and it is worth reaching.

References

Abeles, M. and Goldstein, M. H. (1972). Responses of single units in the primary auditory cortex of the cat to tones and to tone pairs. *Brain Research*, **42**, 337–52.

American Standards Association (1960). *Acoustical Terminology*, SI. 1–1960, American Standards Association, New York.

Anderson, C. M. B. and Whittle, L. S. (1971). Physiological noise and the missing 6 dB. *Acustica*, **24**, 261–72.

Arthur, R. M., Pfeiffer, R. R. and Suga, N. (1971). Properties of 'two-tone inhibition' in primary auditory neurones. *J. Physiol.*, **212**, 593–609.

Attneave, F. and Olson, R. K. (1971). Pitch as a medium: a new approach to psychophysical scaling. *Am. J. Psychol.*, **84**, 147–66.

Bailey, P. J. (1973). Perceptual adaptation for acoustic features in speech. *Speech Perception*, ser. 2, no. 2, 29–34 (Dept. of Psychology, Queen's University of Belfast).

Bailey, P. J. (1974). Procedural variables in speech adaptation. *Speech Perception*, ser. 2, no. 3, 27–34 (Dept. of Psychology, Queen's University of Belfast).

Batteau, D. W. (1967). The role of the pinna in human localization. *Proc. Roy. Soc.* B, **168**, 158–80.

Batteau, D. W. (1968). Listening with the naked ear. In *Neuropsychology of Spatially Oriented Behavior* (ed. S. J. Freedman), Dorsey Press, Illinois.

Bauer, B. B., Torick, E. L. and Allen, R. G. (1971). The measurement of Loudness Level. *J. Accoust. Soc. Am.*, **50**, 405–14.

Beckett, P. and Haggard, M. P. (1973). The psychoacoustical specification of 'tone deafness'. *Speech Perception*, ser. 2, no. 2, 17–22 (Dept. of Psychology, Queen's University of Belfast).

References

Békésy, G. von (1928). Zur theorie des hörens; die schwingungsform der basilarmembran. *Phys. Z.*, **29**, 793–810.

Békésy, G. von (1942). Über die schwingungen der schneckentrennwand beim präparet und ohrenmodell. *Akust. Z.*, **7**, 173–86.

Békésy, G. von (1947). The variation of phase along the basilar membrane with sinusoidal vibrations. *J. Acoust. Soc. Am.* **19**, 452–60.

Békésy, G. von (1960). *Experiments in Hearing* (trans. and ed. E. G. Wever), McGraw-Hill, New York.

Békésy, G. von. (1961). Concerning the fundamental component of periodic pulse patterns and modulated vibrations observed on the cochlear model with nerve supply. *J. Acoust. Soc. Am.*, **33**, 888–96.

Békésy, G. von (1963). Three experiments concerned with pitch perception. *J. Acoust. Soc. Am.*, **35**, 602–6.

Békésy, G. von and Rosenblith, W. A. (1951). The mechanical properties of the ear. In *Handbook of Experimental Psychology* (ed. S. S. Stevens), Wiley, New York.

Beranek, L. L. (1962). *Music, Acoustics and Architecture*, Wiley, New York.

Bilger, R. C. and Feldman, R. M. (1968). Frequency dependence in temporal integration. *76th Meeting of the Acoustical Society of America*, paper A1.

Billone, M. and Raynor, S. (1973). Transmission of radial shear forces to cochlear hair cells. *J. Acoust. Soc. Am.*, **54**, 1143–56.

Bilsen, F. A. (1973). On the influence of the number and phase of harmonics on the perceptibility of the pitch of complex signals. *Acustica*, **28**, 60–5.

Bilsen, F. A. and Goldstein, J. L. (1974). Pitch of dichotically delayed noise and its possible spectral basis. *J. Acoust. Soc. Am.*, **55**, 292–6.

Bilsen, F. A. and Ritsma, R. J. (1967). Repetition pitch mediated by temporal fine structure at dominant spectral regions. *Acustica*, **19**, 114–16.

Blauert, J. (1969/1970). Sound localization in the median plan. *Acustica*, **22**, 206–13.

Boer, E. de (1969a). Reverse correlation. II. Initiation of nerve impulses in the inner ear. *Proc. K. Ned. Akad. Wet.*, **72**, ser. C, 129–51.

Boer, E. de (1969b). Encoding of frequency information in the discharge pattern of auditory nerve fibres. *Int. Audiol.*, **8**, 547.

Boomsliter, P. and Creel, W. (1961). The long pattern hypothesis in harmony and hearing. *J. Music Theory*, **5**, 2–31.

References

Boomsliter, P. and Creel, W. (1963). Extended reference: an unrecognized dynamic in melody. *J. Music Theory*, **7**, 2–22.

Boone, M. M. (1973). Loudness measurements on pure tone and broad band impulsive sounds. *Acustica*, **29**, 198–204.

Bray, D. A., Dirks, D. D. and Morgan, D. E. (1973). Perstimulatory Loudness Adaptation. *J. Acoust. Soc. Am.*, **53**, 1544–8.

Bredberg, G. (1968). Cellular pattern and nerve supply of the human organ of Corti. *Acta Otolaryngol.* Suppl., **236**.

Bregman, A. S. and Campbell, J. (1971). Primary auditory stream segregation and perception of order in rapid sequences of tones. *J. Exp. Psychol.*, **89**, 244–9.

Bregman, A. S. and Dannenbring, G. L. (1973). The effect of continuity on auditory stream segregation. *Percept. Psychophys.*, **13**, 308–12.

Broadbent, D. E. (1958). *Perception and Communication*, Pergamon, London.

Broadbent, D. E. (1967). Word frequency effect and response bias. *Psychol. Rev.*, **74**, 1–15.

Broadbent, D. E. and Gregory, M. (1964). Accuracy of recognition for speech presented to the right and left ears. *Q. J. Exp. Psychol.*, **16**, 359–60.

Broadbent, D. E. and Ladefoged, P. C. (1957). On the fusion of sounds reaching different sense organs. *J. Acoust. Soc. Am.*, **29**, 708–10.

Brugge, J. F., Anderson, D. J., Hind, J. E. and Rose, J. E. (1969). Time structure of discharges in single auditory nerve fibres of the Squirrel Monkey in response to complex periodic sounds. *J. Neurophysiol.*, **32**, 386–401.

Brugge, J. F. and Merzenich, M. M. (1973). Responses of neurones in auditory cortex of macaque monkey to monaural and binaural stimulation. *J. Neurophysiol.*, **36**, 1138–58.

Butler, R. A. (1969). Monaural and binaural localization of noise bursts vertically in the median sagittal plane. *J. Aud. Res.*, **3**, 230–5.

Butler, R. A. (1971). The monaural localisation of tonal stimuli. *Percept. Psychophys.*, **9**, 99–101.

Butterfield, E. C. and Siperstein, G. N. (1970). Influence of contingent auditory stimulation upon non-nutritional suckle. Paper presented at *Third Symposium on Oral Sensation and Perception: The Mouth of the Infant*. To be published by C. C. Thomas, Springfield, Ill.

279

References

Byrne, D. and Dermody, P. (1975). Localization of sound with binaural body-worn hearing aids. *Br. J. Audiol.*, **9**, 107–15.

Carhart, R., Tillman, T. W. and Greetis. (1969). Release from multiple maskers: effects of interaural time disparities. *J. Acoust. Soc. Am.*, **45**, 411–18.

Carter, N. L. (1972). Effects of rise time and repetition rate on the loudness of acoustic transients. *J. Sound Vib.*, **21**, 227–39.

Carterette, E. C., Friedman, M. P. and Lovell, J. D. (1969). Mach bands in hearing. *J. Acoust. Soc. Am.*, **45**, 986–98.

Christman, R. J. and Victor, G. (1955). The perception of direction as a function of binaural temporal and amplitude disparity. Rome Air Development Center ARDC, USAF, Tech. Note RADC-TH-55-302.

Clack, T. D., Erdreich, J. and Knighton, R. W. (1972). Aural harmonics: the monaural phase effects at 1500 Hz, 2000 Hz, and 2500 Hz observed in tone-on-tone masking when $f_1 = 1000$ Hz. *J. Acoust. Soc. Am.*, **52**, 536–41.

Cole, R. A. and Scott, B. (1974). Towards a theory of speech perception. *Psychol. Rev.*, **81**, 348–74.

Coleman, P. D. (1962). Failure to localize the source distance of an unfamiliar sound. *J. Acoust. Soc. Am.*, **34**, 345–6.

Coleman, P. D. (1963). An analysis of cues to auditory depth perception in free space. *Psychol. Bull.*, **60**, 302–15.

Cooper, W. E. (1974). Perceptuomotor adaptation to a speech feature. *Percept. Psychophys.*, **16**, 229–34.

Corliss, E. L. R. (1967). Mechanistic aspects of hearing. *J. Acoust. Soc. Am.*, **41**, 1500–16.

Corliss, E. L. R. and Winzer, G. E. (1964). Study of methods of estimating loudness. *J. Acoust. Soc. Am.*, **38**, 424–8.

Cotzin, M. and Dallenbach, K. M. (1950). 'Facial vision': The role of pitch and loudness in perception of obstacles by the blind. *Am. J. Psychol.*, **63**, 485–515.

Cuddy, L. L. (1968). Practice effects in the absolute judgment of pitch. *J. Acoust. Soc. Am.*, **43**, 1069–76.

Cutting, J. E. and Rosner, B. S. (1974). Categories and boundaries in speech and music. *Percept. Psychophys.*, **16**, 564–70.

Dadson, R. S. and King, J. H. (1952). A determination of the normal threshold of hearing and its relation to the standardization of audiometers. *J. Laryngol. Otol.*, **66**, 366–78.

References

Dallos, P., Billone, M. C., Durrant, J. D., Wang, C.-y. and Raynor, S. (1972). Cochlear inner and outer hair cells: functional differences. *Science, N.Y.*, **177**, 356–8.

Darwin, C. J. (1971). Dichotic backward masking of complex sounds. *Q. J. Exp. Psychol.*, **23**, 386–92.

Darwin, C. J. and Baddely, A. D. (1974). Acoustic memory and the perception of speech. *Cognitive Psychol.*, **6**, 41–60.

Deatherage, B. H. and Evans, T. R. (1969). Binaural masking: backward, forward and simultaneous effects. *J. Acoust. Soc. Am.*, **46**, 362–71.

Deatherage, B. H. and Hirsh, I. J. (1957). Auditory localization of clicks. *J. Acoust. Soc. Am.*, **29**, 132–7.

Dirks, D. and Bower, D. (1970). Effects of forward and backward masking on speech intelligibility. *J. Acoust. Soc. Am.*, **47**, 1003–8.

Divenyi, P. L. and Hirsh, I. J. (1974). Identification of temporal order in three-tone sequences. *J. Acoust. Soc. Am.*, **56**, 144–51.

Dix, M. R. and Hood, J. D. (1973). Symmetrical hearing loss in brain stem lesions. *Acta Otolaryngol.*, **75**, 165–77.

Djupesland, G. and Zwislocki, J. J. (1972). Sound pressure distribution in the outer ear. *Scand. Audiol.*, **1**, 197–203.

Dolan, T. R. and Trahiotis, C. (1972). Binaural interaction in backward masking. *Percept. Psychophys.*, **11**, 92–4.

Dowling, W. J. (1968). Rhythmic fission and perceptual organization. *J. Acoust. Soc. Am.*, **44**, 369.

Dowling, W. J. (1973). The perception of interleaved melodies. *Cognitive Psychol.*, **5**, 322–37.

Duifhuis, H. (1971). Audibility of high harmonics in a periodic pulse II. Time effect. *J. Acoust. Soc. Am.*, **49**, 1155–62.

Duifhuis, H. (1972). *Perceptual Analysis of Sound*, Doctoral dissertation, Eindhoven University of Technology.

Duifhuis, H. (1973). Consequences of peripheral frequency selectivity for nonsimultaneous masking. *J. Acoust. Soc. Am.*, **54**, 1471–88.

Duifhuis, H. (1976). Cochlear nonlinearity and second filter: possible mechanism and implications. *J. Acoust. Soc. Am.*, **59**, 408–23.

Durlach, N. I. (1963). Equalization and cancellation theory of binaural masking level differences. *J. Acoust. Soc. Am.*, **35**, 1206–18.

Durlach, N. I. (1972). Binaural signal detection: equalization and cancellation theory. In *Foundations of Modern Auditory Theory*, vol. II (ed. J. V. Tobias), Academic Press, New York.

References

Egan, J. P. and Hake, H. W. (1950). On the masking pattern of a simple auditory stimulus. *J. Acoust. Soc. Am.*, **22**, 622–30.

Eimas, P. D., Cooper, W. E. and Corbit, J. D. (1973). Some properties of linguistic feature detectors. *Percept. Psychophys.*, **13**, 247–52.

Eimas, P. D. and Corbit, J. D. (1973). Selective adaptation of linguistic feature detectors. *Cognitive Psychol.*, **4**, 99–109.

Elliot, D. N. and Fraser, W. R. (1970). Fatigue and adaptation. In *Foundations of Modern Auditory Theory*, vol. I (ed. J. V. Tobias), Academic Press, New York.

Elliot, D. N., Stein, L. and Harrison, M. J. (1960). Determination of absolute-intensity thresholds and frequency-difference thresholds in cats. *J. Acoust. Soc. Am.*, **32**, 380–84.

Elliot, L. L. (1962). Backward and forward masking of probe tones of different frequencies. *J. Acoust. Soc. Am.*, **34**, 1116–17.

Elliot, L. L. (1967). Development of auditory narrow-band frequency contours. *J. Acoust. Soc. Am.*, **42**, 143–53.

Eliot, L. L. (1969). Masking of tones before, during, and after brief silent periods in noise. *J. Acoust. Soc. Am.*, **45**, 1277–9.

Elliot, L. L. (1971). Backward and forward masking. *Audiology*, **10**, 65–76.

Evans, E. F. (1968). Cortical Representation. In *Hearing Mechanisms in Vertebrates* (ed. A. V. S. de Reuck and J. Knight), Churchill, London.

Evans, E. F. (1975). The sharpening of cochlear frequency selectivity in the normal and abnormal cochlea. *Audiology*, **14**, 419–42.

Evans, E. F. and Palmer, A. R. (1975). Responses of units in the cochlear nerve and nucleus of the cat to signals in the presence of bandstop noise. *J. Physiol.*, **252**, 60–62P.

Exner, S. (1876). Zur lehre von den gehorsempfindungen. *Pflügers Archiv*, **13**, 228–53.

Fant, C. G. M. (1960). *Acoustic Theory of Speech Production*, Mouton, The Hague.

Fant, C. G. M. (1963). Comments on 'A motor theory of speech perception' by A. M. Lieberman, F. S. Cooper, K. S. Harris and P. F. Macneilage. In *Proceedings of the Speech Communication Seminar*, vol. 3 (ed. C. G. M. Fant), Royal Institute of Technology, Stockholm.

Feldtkeller, R. and Zwicker, E. (1956). *Das Ohr als Nachrichtenempfänger*, S. Hirzel, Stuttgart.

References

Fellgett, P. B. (1974). Ambisonic reproduction of directionality in surround-sound systems. *Nature*, **252**, 534-8.

Feth, L. L. (1972). Combinations of amplitude and frequency difference in auditory discrimination. *Acustica*, **26**, 67-77.

Fischer-Jørgensen, E. (1972). Tape cutting experiments with Danish stop consonants in initial position. Ann. Rep. VII, University of Copenhagen, Institute of Phonetics.

Fletcher, H. (1940). Auditory patterns. *Rev. Mod. Phys.*, **12**, 47-65.

Fourcin, A. J. (1970). Central pitch and auditory lateralization. In *Frequency Analysis and Periodicity Detection in Hearing* (ed. R. Plomp and G. F. Smoorenburg), A. W. Sijthoff, Leiden.

Fourcin, A. J. (1975). Speech perception in the absence of speech productive ability. In *Language, Cognitive Defects and Retardation* (ed. N. O'Conner), Butterworths, London.

Freedman, S. J. and Fisher, H. G. (1968). The role of the pinna in auditory localization. In *Neuropsychology of Spatially Oriented Behavior* (ed. S. J. Freedman), Dorsey Press, Illinois.

Freedman, S. J., Wilson, L. and Rekosh, J. H. (1967). Compensation for auditory re-arrangement in hand-ear coordination. *Percept. Motor Skills*, **24**, 1207-10.

Gardner, M. B. and Gardner, R. S. (1973). Problem of localization in the median plan: effect of pinnae cavity occlusion. *J. Acoust. Soc. Am.*, **53**, 400-8.

Garner, W. R. and Miller, G. A. (1947). The masked threshold of pure tones as a function of duration. *J. Exp. Psychol.*, **37**, 293-303.

Gässler, G. (1954). Über die hörschwelle für schallereignisse mit verschieden breitem frequenzspektrum. *Acustica*, **4**, 408-14.

Gebhardt, C. J. and Goldstein, D. P. (1972). Frequency discrimination and the M.L.D. *J. Acoust. Soc. Am.*, **51**, 1228-32.

Gerzon, M. A. (1971). Synthetic stereo reverberation. *Studio Sound*, **13**, 632-5.

Gerzon, M. A. (1975). Dummy head recording. *Studio Sound*, **17**, 42-4.

Goldstein, J. L. (1967). Auditory nonlinearity. *J. Acoust. Soc. Am.*, **41**, 676-89.

Goldstein, J. L. (1972). Evidence from aural combination tones and musical tones against classical periodicity theory. In *Hearing Theory 1972*, IPO, Eindhoven, The Netherlands.

References

Goldstein, J. L. (1973). An optimum processor theory for the central formation of the pitch of complex tones. *J. Acoust. Soc. Am.*, **54**, 1496–1516.

Green, D. M. (1973). Temporal acuity as a function of frequency. *J. Acoust. Soc. Am.*, **54**, 373–9.

Green, D. M., Birdsall, T. G. and Tanner, W. P. (1957). Signal detection as a function of signal intensity and duration. *J. Acoust. Soc. Am.*, **29**, 523–31.

Greenwood, D. D. (1961). Auditory masking and the critical band. *J. Acoust. Soc. Am.*, **33**, 484–501.

Groen, J. J. (1964). Super- and subliminal binaural beats. *Acta Otolaryngol.*, **57**, 224–30.

Gruber, J. and Boerger, G. (1971). Binaurale verdeckungspegeldifferenzen (BMLD) und vor- und rückwärtsverdeckung. *Proc. 7th Int. Congr. on Acoustics, Budapest*, paper 23H5.

Hafter, E. R. and Carrier, S. C. (1972). Binaural interaction in low-frequency stimuli: the inability to trade time and intensity completely. *J. Acoust. Soc. Am.*, **51**, 1852–62.

Hafter, E. R. and Jeffress, L. A. (1968). Two-image lateralization of tones and clicks. *J. Acoust. Soc. Am.*, **44**, 563–9.

Haggard, M. P. (1974). Feasibility of rapid critical bandwidth estimates. *J. Acoust. Soc. Am.*, **55**, 304–8.

Haggard, M. P. and Bates, J. (1974). Changes in auditory perception in the menstrual cycle. *Speech Perception*, ser. 2, no. 3, 55–74 (Department of Psychology, Queen's University of Belfast).

Hamilton, P. M. (1957). Noise masked thresholds as a function of tonal duration and masking noise band width. *J. Acoust. Soc. Am.*, **29**, 506–11.

Handel, S. (1973). Temporal segmentation of repeating auditory patterns. *J. Exp. Psychol.*, **101**, 46–54.

Hansen, V. and Madsen, E. R. (1974). On aural phase detection. *J. Audio Engng. Soc.*, **22**, 10–14.

Harris, G. G. (1960). Binaural interactions of impulsive stimuli and pure tones. *J. Acoust. Soc. Am.*, **32**, 685–92.

Harris, J. D. (1963). Loudness discrimination. *J. Speech Hear. Dis. Monogr. Suppl.* **11**, 1–63.

Harris, J. D. (1972). Audition. *Ann. Rev. Psychol.*, **23**, 313–46.

Harris, J. D. and Sergeant, R. L. (1971). Monaural/binaural minimum audible angles for a moving sound source. *J. Speech Hear. Res.*, **14**, 618–29.

References

Hawkins, J. E. and Stevens, S. S. (1950). The masking of pure tones and of speech by white noise. *J. Acoust. Soc. Am.*, **22**, 6–13.

Held, R. (1955). Shifts in binaural localization after prolonged exposures to atypical combination of stimuli. *Am. J. Psychol.*, **68**, 526–48.

Helmholtz, H. L. F. von (1863). *Die Lehre von den Tonempfindungen als physiologische Grundlage für die Theorie der Musik*, 1st edn, F. Vieweg Braunschweig.

Henning, G. B. (1966). Frequency discrimination of random amplitude tones. *J. Acoust. Soc. Am.*, **39**, 336–9.

Henning, G. B. (1967). A model for auditory discrimination and detection. *J. Acoust. Soc. Am.*, **42**, 1325–34.

Henning, G. B. (1974). Detectability of interaural delay with high-frequency complex waveforms. *J. Acoust. Soc. Am.*, **55**, 84–90.

Heyes, A. D. and Ferris, A. J. (1975). Auditory localization using hearing aids. *Br. J. Audiol.*, **9**, 102–6.

Hind, J. E. (1972). Physiological correlates of auditory stimulus periodicity. *Audiology*, **11**, 42–57.

Hind, J. E., Rose, J. E., Brugge, J. F. and Anderson, D. J. (1967). Coding of information pertaining to paired low-frequency tones in single auditory nerve fibers of the squirrel monkey. *J. Neurophysiol.*, **30**, 794–816.

Hirsh, I. J. (1950). The relation between localization and intelligibility. *J. Acoust. Soc. Am.*, **22**, 196–200.

Hirsh, I. J. (1959). Auditory perception of temporal order. *J. Acoust. Soc. Am.*, **31**, 759–67.

Hirsh, I. J. (1971). Masking of speech and auditory localization. *Audiology*, **10**, 110–14.

Hirsh, I. J. and Bilger, R. C. (1955). Auditory-threshold recovery after exposures to pure tones. *J. Acoust. Soc. Am.*, **27**, 1186–94.

Hirsh, I. J. and Ward, W. D. (1952). Recovery of the auditory threshold after strong acoustic stimulation. *J. Acoust. Soc. Am.*, **24**, 131–41.

Hood, J. D. (1950). Studies in auditory fatigue and adaptation. *Acta Otolaryngol. Suppl.* 92.

Hood, J. D. (1972). Fundamentals of identification of sensorineural hearing loss. *Sound*, **6**, 21–6.

House, A. S., Stevens, K. N., Sandel, T. T. and Arnold, J. B. (1962). On the learning of speechlike vocabularies. *J. Verb. Learn. Verb. Behav.*, **1**, 133–43.

References

Houtgast, T. (1972). Psychophysical evidence for lateral inhibition in hearing. *J. Acoust. Soc. Am.*, **51**, 1885–94.

Houtsma, A. J. M. and Goldstein, J. L. (1972). The central origin of the pitch of complex tones: evidence from musical interval recognition. *J. Acoust. Soc. Am.*, **51**, 520–9.

Howes, W. L. (1971). Loudness determined by power summation. *Acustica*, **25**, 343–9.

Hubel, D. H. and Wiesel, T. N. (1968). Receptive fields and functional architecture of monkey striate cortex. *J. Physiol.*, **195**, 215–43.

Huggins, W. H. and Cramer, E. M. (1958). Creation of pitch through binaural interaction. *J. Acoust. Soc. Am.*, **30**, 413–17.

Huggins, W. H. and Licklider, J. C. R. (1951). Place mechanisms of auditory frequency analysis. *J. Acoust. Soc. Am.*, **23**, 290–9.

Hughes, J. R. and Rosenblith, W. A. (1957). Electrophysiological evidence for auditory sensitization. *J. Acoust. Soc. Am.*, **29**, 275–80.

Hughes, J. W. (1946). The threshold of audition for short periods of stimulation. *Proc. Roy. Soc.* B, **133**, 486–90.

Hyde, S. R. (1972). Automatic speech recognition: a critical survey of the literature. In *Human Communication: A Unified View* (ed. E. E. David and P. B. Denes), McGraw-Hill, New York.

Jacobs, J. E. and Wittman, P. (1964). Psychoacoustics, the determining factor in stereo disc recording. *J. Audio Engng. Soc.*, **12**, 115–23.

Javel, E. (1974). Discharge patterns of auditory nerve of chinchilla to AM tones possessing low subjective pitch. *J. Acoust. Soc. Am.*, **55**, Suppl. S85.

Jeffress, L. A. (1964). Stimulus-oriented approach to detection. *J. Acust. Soc. Am.*, **36**, 766–74.

Jeffress, L. A. (1971). Detection and lateralization of binaural signals. *Audiology*, **10**, 77–84.

Jerger, J. F. (1957). Auditory adaptation. *J. Acoust. Soc. Am.*, **29**, 357–63.

Johnson, D. L. and Gierke, H. von (1974). Audibility of infrasound. *J. Acoust. Soc. Am.*, **56**, Suppl., S37.

Johnstone, B. M. and Boyle, A. J. F. (1967). Basilar membrane vibration examined with the Mössbauer technique. *Science, N.Y.*, **158**, 389–90.

Johnstone, B. M. and Sellick, P. M. (1972). The peripheral auditory apparatus. *Q. Rev. Biophys.*, **5**, 1–57.

286

References

Johnstone, B. M., Taylor, K. J. and Boyle, A. J. (1970). Mechanics of guinea-pig cochlea. *J. Acoust. Soc. Am.*, **47**, 504–9.

Kalil, R. and Freedman, S. J. (1967). Compensation for auditory re-arrangement in the absence of observer movements. *Percept. Motor Skills*, **24**, 475–8.

Karlan, M. S., Tonndorf, J. and Khanna, S. M. (1972). Dual origin of cochlear microphonics: inner and outer hair cells. *Ann. Otol. Rhinol. Laryngol.*, **81**, 696–705.

Katz, S. J. and Berry, R. C. (1971). Speech modulated noise. Paper presented at the *81st Meeting of the Acoustical Society of America*.

Kay, L. (1966). Spectacles for the blind. In *Sensory Devices for the Blind*, St. Dunstan's, London.

Kay, R. H. and Matthews, D. R. (1972). On the existence in human auditory pathways of channels selectively tuned to the modulation present in frequency modulated sounds. *J. Physiol.*, **225**, 657–77.

Kellog, W. N. (1962). Sonar system of the blind. *Science, N.Y.*, **137**, 399–404.

Kiang, N.Y.-S. (1968). A survey of recent developments in the study of auditory physiology. *Ann. Otol. Rhinol. Laryngol.*, **77**, 656–75.

Kiang, N. Y.-S., Watanabe, T., Thomas, E. C. and Clark, L. F. (1965). *Discharge Patterns of Single Fibers in the Cat's Auditory Nerve*, M.I.T.Press, Cambridge, Mass.

Kimura, D. (1961). Some effects of temporal lobe damage on auditory perception. *Can. J. Psychol.*, **15**, 156–65.

Kimura, D. (1964). Left–right differences in the perception of melodies. *Q. J. Exp. Psychol.*, **16**, 355–8.

Klump, R. G. and Eady, H. R. (1956). Some measurements of inter-aural time difference thresholds. *J. Acoust. Soc. Am.*, **28**, 859–60.

Kohllöffel, L. U. E. (1972). A study of basilar membrane vibrations II. The vibratory amplitude and phase pattern along the basilar membrane (post-mortem). *Acustica*, **27**, 66–81.

Kruskal, J. B. (1964). Nonmetric multidimensional scaling: a numeri-cal method. *Psychometrika*, **29**, 115–29.

Kuyper, P. (1972). The cocktail party effect. *Audiology*, **11**, 277–82.

Kuyper, P. and de Boer, E. (1969). Evaluation of stereophonic fitting of hearing aids to hard-of-hearing children. *Int. Audiol.*, **8**, 524–8.

Ladefoged, P. and Broadbent, D. E. (1960). Perception of sequence in auditory events. *Q. J. Exp. Psychol.*, **12**, 162–70.

Lamore, P. J. J. (1972). Perception of octave complexes. In *Hearing Theory 1972*, IPO, Eindhoven, The Netherlands.

Lane, H. L. (1965). The motor theory of speech perception: a critical review. *Psychol. Rev.*, **72**, 275–309.

Legouix, J. P., Remond, M. C. and Greenbaum, H. B. (1973). Interference and two-tone inhibition. *J. Acoust. Soc. Am.*, **53**, 409–19.

Lenneberg, E. (1962). Understanding language without ability to speak: a case report. *J. Abnorm. Soc. Psychol.*, **65**, 419–25.

Liberman, A. M. (1957). Some results of research on speech perception. *J. Acoust. Soc. Am.*, **28**, 117–23.

Liberman, A. M., Cooper, E. S., Harris, K. S. and Macneilage, P. F. (1963). A motor theory of speech perception. In *Proceedings of Speech Communication Seminar*, vol. 3 (ed. C. G. M. Fant), Royal Institute of Technology, Stockholm.

Liberman, A. M., Cooper, F. S., Shankweiler, D. P. and Studdert-Kennedy, M. (1967). Perception of the speech code. *Psychol. Rev.*, **74**, 431–61.

Licklider, J. C. R. (1956). Auditory frequency analysis. In *Information Theory* (ed. C. Cherry), Academic Press, New York.

Licklider, J. C. R., Webster, J. C. and Hedlun, J. M. (1950). On the frequency limits of binaural beats. *J. Acoust. Soc. Am.*, **22**, 468–73.

Lindqvist, J. and Sundberg, J. (1971). Perception of the octave interval. *7th Int. Congr. on Acoustics, Budapest*, paper 20 S 12.

Locke, S. and Kellar, L. (1973). Categorical perception in a non-linguistic mode. *Cortex*, **9**, 353–69.

McFadden, D., Jeffress, L. A. and Ermey, H. L. (1971). Differences of interaural phase and lefel in detection and lateralization: 250 Hz. *J. Acoust. Soc. Am.*, **50**, 1484–93.

McFadden, D., Jeffress, L. A. and Ermey, H. L. (1972). Differences of interaural phase and level in detection and lateralization: 1000 and 2000 Hz. *J. Acoust. Soc. Am.*, **52**, 1197–206.

McGill, W. J. and Goldberg, J. P. (1968a). A study of the near-miss involving Weber's law and pure-tone intensity discrimination. *Percept. Psychophys.*, **4**, 105–9.

McGill, W. J. and Goldberg, J. P. (1968b). Pure-tone intensity discrimination and energy detection. *J. Acoust. Soc. Am.*, **44**, 576–81.

Maiwald, D. (1967). Die berechnung von modulationsschwellen mit hilfe eines functionsschemas. *Acustica*, **18**, 193–207.

Mayer, A. M. (1894). Researches in acoustics. *Lond. Edinb. Dubl. Phil. Mag.*, **37**, ser. 5, 259–88.

References

Mersenne, M. (1636). *Traite des Instrumens*, Book IV, Sebastian Cramoisy, Paris.

Merzenich, M. M., Knight, P. L. and Roth, G. L. (1973a). Cochleotopic organization of primary auditory cortex in the cat. *Brain Res.*, **63**, 343–6.

Merzenich, M. M., Michelson, R. P., Schindler, R. A., Pettit, C. R. and Reid, M. (1973b). Neural encoding of sound sensation evoked by electrical stimulation of the acoustic nerve. *Ann. Otol.*, **82**, 486–503.

Merzenich, M. M., Schindler, D. N. and White, M. W. (1974). Symposium on cochlear implants. II. Feasibility of multichannel scala tympani stimulation. *Laryngoscope*, **84**, 1887–93.

Meyer, M. (1898). Zur theorie der differenztöne und der gehörsempfindungen überhaupt. *Beitr. Akust. Musikwiss.*, **2**, 25–65.

Miller, G. A. (1947). Sensitivity to changes in the intensity of white noise and its relation to masking and loudness. *J. Acoust. Soc. Am.*, **19**, 609–19.

Miller, G. A. and Taylor, W. (1948). The perception of repeated bursts of noise. *J. Acoust. Soc. Am.*, **20**, 171–82.

Miller, J. D. (1974). Effects of noise on people. *J. Acoust. Soc. Am.*, **56**, 729–64.

Mills, A. W. (1960). Lateralization of high-frequency tones. *J. Acoust. Soc. Am.*, **32**, 132–4.

Mills, A. W. (1972). Auditory localization. In *Foundations of Modern Auditory Theory*, vol. II (ed. J. V. Tobias), Academic Press, New York.

Møller, A. R. (1972). Coding of sounds in lower levels of the auditory system. *Q. Rev. Biophys.*, **5**, 59–155.

Mollon, J. (1974). After-effects and the brain. *New Scientist*, 21st Feb., 479–82.

Moore, B. C. J. (1972). Some experiments relating to the perception of pure tones: possible clinical applications. *Sound*, **6**, 73–9.

Moore, B. C. J. (1973a). Frequency difference limens for short-duration tones. *J. Acoust. Soc. Am.*, **54**, 610–19.

Moore, B. C. J. (1973b). Frequency difference limens for narrow bands of noise. *J. Acoust. Soc. Am.*, **54**, 888–96.

Moore, B. C. J. (1973c). Some experiments relating to the perception of complex tones. *Q. J. Exp. Psychol.*, **25**, 451–75.

Moore, B. C. J. (1974). Relation between the critical bandwidth and the frequency-difference limen. *J. Acoust. Soc. Am.*, **55**, 359.

References

Moore, B. C. J. and Raab, D. H. (1974). Pure-tone intensity discrimination: some experiments relating to the 'near-miss' to Weber's law. *J. Acoust. Soc. Am.*, **55**, 1049–54.

Moore, B. C. J. and Raab, D. H. (1975). Intensity discrimination for noise bursts in the presence of a continuous, bandstop background: effects of level, width of the bandstop, and duration. *J. Acoust. Soc. Am.*, **57**, 400–5.

Moore, T. J. and Welsh, J. R. (1970). Forward and backward enhancement of sensitivity in the auditory system. *J. Acoust. Soc. Am.*, **47**, 534–9.

Morton, J. (1964). A model for continuous language behaviour. *Language and Speech*, **7**, 40–70.

Mulligan, B., Mulligan, M. and Stonecypher, J. F. (1967). Critical band in binaural detection. *J. Acoust. Soc. Am.*, **41**, 7–12.

Newman, E. B. (1948). Chapter 14 in *Foundations of Psychology* (ed. E. G. Boring, H. S. Langfeld and H. P. Weld), Wiley, New York.

Noorden, L. P. A. S. van (1971). Rhythmic fission as a function of tone rate. *IPO Annual Progress Rep.*, **6**, 9–12, Eindhoven, The Netherlands.

Nordmark, J. O. (1970). Time and frequency analysis. In *Foundations of Modern Auditory Theory*, vol. I (ed. J. V. Tobias), Academic Press, New York.

Ohm, G. S. (1843). Ueber die definition des tones, nebst daran geknüpfter theorie der sirene und ähnlicher tonbildender vorrichtungen. *Ann. Phys. Chem.*, **59**, 513–65.

Olsen, W. O. and Carhart, R. (1966). Integration of acoustic power at threshold by normal hearers. *J. Acoust. Soc. Am.*, **40**, 591–9.

Patterson, J. H. (1971). Additivity of forward and backward masking as a function of signal frequency. *J. Acoust. Soc. Am.*, **50**, 1123–5.

Patterson, J. H. and Green, D. M. (1970). Discrimination of transient signals having identical energy spectra. *J. Acoust. Soc. Am.*, **48**, 894–905.

Patterson, R. D. (1974). Auditory filter shape. *J. Acoust. Soc. Am.*, **55**, 802–9.

Patterson, R. D. (1976). Auditory filter shapes derived with noise stimuli. *J. Acoust. Soc. Am.*, **59**, 640–54.

Peiper, A. (1963). *Cerebral Function in Infancy and Childhood*, Consultants Bureau, New York.

References

Pisoni, D. B. (1973). Auditory and phonetic memory codes in the discrimination of consonants and vowels. *Percept. Psychophys.*, **13**, 253–60.

Plenge, G. (1972). Über das problem der im-kopf-lokalisation. *Acustica*, **26**, 213–21.

Plenge, G. (1974). On the differences between localization and lateralization. *J. Acoust. Soc. Am.*, **56**, 944–51.

Plomp, R. (1964). The ear as a frequency analyser. *J. Acoust. Soc. Am.*, **36**, 1628–36.

Plomp, R. (1965). Detectability threshold for combination tones. *J. Acoust. Soc. Am.*, **37**, 1110–23.

Plomp, R. (1967). Pitch of complex tones. *J. Acoust. Soc. Am.*, **41**, 1526–33.

Plomp, R. (1968). Pitch, timbre and hearing theory. *Int. Audiol.*, **7**, 322–44.

Plomp, R. (1970). Timbre as a multidimensional attribute of complex tones. In *Frequency Analysis and Periodicity Detection in Hearing* (ed. R. Plomp and G. F. Smoorenburg), Sijtthoff, Leiden.

Plomp, R. and Bouman, M. A. (1959). Relation between hearing threshold and duration for tone pulses. *J. Acoust. Soc. Am.*, **31**, 749–58.

Plomp, R. and Levelt, W. J. M. (1965). Tonal consonance and critical bandwidth. *J. Acoust. Soc. Am.*, **38**, 548–60.

Plomp, R., Pols, L. C. W. and Geer, J. P. van de (1967). Dimensional analysis of vowel spectra. *J. Acoust. Soc. Am.*, **41**, 707–12.

Plomp, R. and Steeneken, H. J. M. (1969). Effect of phase on the timbre of complex tones. *J. Acoust. Soc. Am.*, **46**, 409–21.

Pollack, I. (1952). The information of elementary auditory displays. *J. Acoust. Soc. Am.*, **24**, 745–9.

Pollack, I. (1969). Periodicity pitch for white noise—fact or artifact. *J. Acoust. Soc. Am.*, **45**, 237–8.

Pols, L. C. W., Kamp., L. J. Th. van der and Plomp, R. (1969). Perceptual and physical space of vowel sounds. *J. Acoust. Soc. Am.*, **46**, 458–67.

Port, E. (1963). Uber die lautstärke einzelner kurzer schallimpulse. *Acustica*, **13**, 212–23.

Potter, R. K., Kopp, G. A. and Green, H. C. (1947). *Visible Speech*, Van Nostrand, New York.

Raiford, C. A. and Schubert, E. D. (1971). Recognition of phase changes in octave complexes. *J. Acoust. Soc. Am.*, **50**, 559–67.

References

Rainbolt, H. and Small, A. M. (1972). Mach bands in auditory masking: an attempted replication. *J. Acoust. Soc. Am.*, **51**, 567–74.

Rakowski, A. (1972). Direct comparison of absolute and relative pitch. In *Hearing Theory 1972*, IPO Eindhoven, The Netherlands.

Rhode, W. S. (1971). Observations of the vibration of the basilar membrane in squirrel monkeys using the Mössbauer technique. *J. Acoust. Soc. Am.*, **49**, 1218–31.

Rhode, W. S. and Robles, L. (1974). Evidence from Mössbauer experiments for non-linear vibration in the cochlea. *J. Acoust. Soc. Am.*, **55**, 588–96.

Rice, C. E. (1967). Human echo perception. *Science, N.Y.*, **155**, 656–64.

Riesz, R. R. (1928). Differential intensity sensitivity of the ear for pure tones. *Phys. Rev.*, **31** (ser. 2), 867–75.

Ritsma, R. J. (1962). Existence region of the tonal residue. I. *J. Acoust. Soc. Am.*, **34**, 1224–9.

Ritsma, R. J. (1963). Existence region of the tonal residue. II. *J. Acoust. Soc. Am.*, **35**, 1241–5.

Ritsma, R. J. (1967a). Frequencies dominant in the perception of the pitch of complex sounds. *J. Acoust. Soc. Am.*, **42**, 191–8.

Ritsma, R. J. (1967b). Frequencies dominant in the perception of periodic pulses of alternating polarity. *IPO Annual Prog. Rep.*, Eindhoven, **2**, 14–24.

Ritsma, R. J. (1970). Periodicity detection. In *Frequency Analysis and Periodicity Detection in Hearing* (ed. R. Plomp and G. F. Smoorenburg), Sijthoff, Leiden.

Robertson, D. (1976). Correspondence between sharp tuning and two-tone inhibition in primary auditory neurones. *Nature*, **259**, 477–8.

Robertson, D. and Manley, G. A. (1974). Manipulation of frequency analysis in the cochlear ganglion of the guinea-pig. *J. Comp. Physiol.*, **91**, 363–75.

Robinson, D. W. and Dadson, R. S. (1956). A redetermination of the equal-loudness relations for pure tones. *Br. J. Appl. Phys.*, **7**, 166–81.

Rodenburg, M. (1972). *Sensitivity of the Auditory System to Differences in Intensity*, Unpublished Ph.D. Thesis, Medical Faculty, Rotterdam.

References

Rose, J. E., Brugge, J. F., Anderson, D. J. and Hind, J. E. (1967). Phase-locked response to low-frequency tones in single auditory nerve fibers of the squirrel monkey. *J. Neurophysiol.*, **30**, 769–93.

Rose, J. E., Brugge, J. F., Anderson, D. J. and Hind, J. E. (1968). Patterns of activity in single auditory nerve fibers of the squirrel monkey. In *Hearing Mechanisms in Vertebrates* (ed. A. V. S. de Reuck and J. Knight), Churchill, London.

Rose, J. E., Hind, J. E., Anderson, D. J. and Brugge, J. F. (1971). Some effects of stimulus intensity on response of auditory nerve fibers in the squirrel monkey. *J. Neurophysiol.*, **34**, 685–99.

Royer, F. L. and Garner, W. R. (1966). Response uncertainty and perceptual difficulty of auditory temporal patterns. *Percept. Psychophys.*, **1**, 41–7.

Royer, F. L. and Garner, W. R. (1970). Perceptual organization of nine-element auditory temporal patterns. *Percept. Psychophys.*, **7**, 115–20.

Ruggero, M. A. (1973). Response to noise of auditory nerve fibers in the squirrel monkey. *J. Neurophysiol.*, **36**, 569–87.

Sachs, M. B. (1971). *Physiology of the Auditory System*, National Educational Consultants, Baltimore.

Sachs, M. B. and Abbas, P. J. (1974). Rate versus level functions for auditory-nerve fibers in cats: tone-burst stimuli. *J. Acoust. Soc. Am.*, **56**, 1835–47.

Sachs, M. B. and Kiang, N.Y.-S. (1968). Two-tone inhibition in auditory-nerve fibers. *J. Acoust. Soc. Am.*, **43**, 1120–8.

Sandel, T. T., Teas, D. C., Feddersen, W. E. and Jeffress, L. A. (1955). Localization of sound from single and paired sources. *J. Acoust. Soc. Am.*, **27**, 842–52.

Schacknow, P. N. and Raab, D. H. (1973). Intensity discrimination of tone bursts and the form of the Weber function. *Percept. Psychophys.*, **14**, 449–50.

Scharf, B. (1961). Complex sounds and critical bands. *Psychol. Bull.*, **58**, 205–17.

Scharf, B. (1970). Critical bands. In *Foundations of Modern Auditory Theory*, vol. I (ed. J. V. Tobias), Academic Press, New York.

Scharf, B. (1971). Fundamentals of auditory masking. *Audiology*, **10**, 30–40.

Schouten, J. F. (1940). The residue and the mechanism of hearing. *Proc. K. Ned. Akad. Wet.*, **43**, 991–9.

References

Schouten, J. F. (1968). The perception of timbre. In *Reports 6th International Congress on Acoustics, Tokyo, Japan*, vol. I, GP–6–2.

Schouten, J. F. (1970). The residue revisited. In *Frequency Analysis and Periodicity Detection in Hearing* (ed. R. Plomp and G. F. Smoorenburg), Sijthoff, Leiden.

Schouten, J. F., Ritsma, R. J. and Cardozo, B. L. (1962). Pitch of the residue. *J. Acoust. Soc. Am.*, **34**, 1418–24.

Schroeder, M. R. and Atal, B. S. (1963). Computer simulation of sound transmission in rooms. *IEEE Int. Conv. Rec.*, **7**, 150–5.

Schroeder, M. R., Gottlob, D. and Siebrasse, K. F. (1974). Comparative study of European concert halls: correlation of subjective preference with geometric and acoustic parameters. *J. Acoust. Soc. Am.*, **56**, 1195–201.

Schubert, E. D. (1969). On estimating aural harmonics. *J. Acoust. Soc. Am.*, **45**, 790–1.

Schuknecht, H. F. (1970). Functional manifestations of lesions of the sensorineural structures. In *Foundations of Modern Auditory Theory*, vol. I (ed. J. V. Tobias), Academic Press, New York.

Shaxby, J. H. and Gage, F. H. (1932). Studies in the localization of sound. Med. Res. Council Spec. Rept. Ser. No. 166, 1–32.

Sheeley, E. C. and Bilger, R. C. (1964). Temporal integration as a function of frequency. *J. Acoust. Soc. Am.*, **36**, 1850–7.

Shepard, R. N. (1962). The analysis of proximities: multidimensional scaling with an unknown distance function. *Psychometrika*, **27**, 125–40.

Shower, E. G. and Biddulph, R. (1931). Differential pitch sensitivity of the ear. *J. Acoust. Soc. Am.*, **2**, 275–87.

Siebert, W. M. (1968). Stimulus transformations in the peripheral auditory system. In *Recognizing Patterns* (ed. P. A. Kolers and M. Eden), M.I.T. Press, Cambridge, Mass.

Siebert, W. M. (1970). Frequency discrimination in the auditory system: place or periodicity mechanisms. *Proc. IEEE*, **58**, 723–30.

Simmons, F. B. (1966). Electrical stimulation of the auditory nerve in man. *Arch. Otolaryngol.*, **84**, 2–54.

Slater, P. (1960). The analysis of personal preferences. *Br. J. Stat. Psychol.*, **8**, 119.

Small, A. M., Boggess, J., Klich, R., Kuehn, D., Thelin, J. and Wiley, T. (1972). MLD's in forward and backward masking. *J. Acoust. Soc. Am.*, **51**, 1365–7.

References

Smoorenburg, G. F. (1970). Pitch perception of two-frequency stimuli. *J. Acoust. Soc. Am.*, **48**, 924–41.

Soderquist, D. R. (1970). Frequency analysis and the critical band. *Psychon. Sci.*, **21**, 117–19.

Soderquist, D. R. and Lindsey, J. W. (1972). Physiological noise as a masker of low frequencies: the cardiac cycle. *J. Acoust. Soc. Am.*, **52**, 1216–20.

Spoendlin, H. (1970). Structural basis of peripheral frequency analysis. In *Frequency Analysis and Periodicity Detection in Hearing* (ed. R. Plomp and G. F. Smoorenburg), Sijthoff, Leiden.

Srinivasan, R. (1971). Auditory critical bandwidth for short duration signals. *J. Acoust. Soc. Am.*, **50**, 616–22.

Stahl, D. (1975). Artificial head stereophony—first application in broadcasting. *SERT Journal*, **9**, 171–3.

Stephens, S. D. G. (1973). Auditory temporal integration as a function of intensity. *J. Sound Vib.*, **30**, 109–26.

Stephens, S. D. G. (1974). Methodological factors influencing loudness of short duration sounds. *J. Sound Vib.*, **37**, 235–46.

Stevens, K. N. (1968). On the relations between speech movements and speech perception. *Z. Phonetik Sprachwiss. Kommunikationsforsch.*, **21**, 102–6.

Stevens, K. N. and House, A. S. (1972). Speech perception. In *Foundations of Modern Auditory Theory*, vol. II (ed. J. V. Tobias), Academic Press, New York.

Stevens, S. S. (1957). On the psychophysical law. *Psychol. Rev.*, **64**, 153–81.

Stevens, S. S. (1972). Perceived level of noise by Mark VII and decibels (E). *J. Acoust. Soc. Am.*, **51**, 575–601.

Stevens, S. S. and Newman, E. B. (1936). The localization of actual sources of sound. *Am. J. Psychol.*, **48**, 297–306.

Sturges, P. T. and Martin, J. F. (1974). Rhythmic structure in auditory temporal pattern perception and immediate memory. *J. Exp. Psychol.*, **102**, 377–83.

Supa, M., Cotzin, M. and Dallenbach, K. M. (1944). 'Facial vision': The perception of obstacles by the blind. *Am. J. Psychol.*, **57**, 133–83.

Swets, J. A., Green, D. M. and Tanner, W. P., Jr. (1962). On the width of critical bands. *J. Acoust. Soc. Am.*, **34**, 108–13.

Tanner, W. P. and Rivette, C. L. (1964). Experimental study of 'tone deafness'. *J. Acoust. Soc. Am.*, **36**, 1465–7.

References

Tanner, W. P. and Sorkin, R. D. (1972). The theory of signal detectability. In *Foundations of Modern Auditory Theory*, vol. II (ed. J. V. Tobias), Academic Press, London.

Tasaki, I. (1954). Nerve impulses in individual auditory nerve fibres of guinea-pig. *J. Neurophysiol.*, 17, 97–122.

Terhardt, E. (1970). Frequency analysis and periodicity detection in the sensations of roughness and periodicity pitch. In *Frequency Analysis and Periodicity Detection in Hearing* (ed. R. Plomp and G. F. Smoorenburg), Sijthoff, Leiden.

Terhardt, E. (1971). Die tonhöhe harmonischer klänge und das oktavintervall. *Acustica*, 24, 126–36.

Terhardt, E. (1972a). Zur tonhöhenwahrnehmung von klängen. I. Psychoakustische grundlagen. *Acustica*, 26, 173–86.

Terhardt, E. (1972b). Zur tonhöhenwahrnehmung von klängen. II. Ein funktionsschema. *Acustica*, 26, 187–99.

Terhardt, E. (1972c). Frequency and time resolution of the ear in pitch perception of complex tones. In *Hearing Theory 1972*, IPO, Eindhoven, The Netherlands.

Terhardt, E. (1974). Pitch, consonance and harmony. *J. Acoust. Soc. Am.*, 55, 1061–9.

Terhardt, E. and Fastl, H. (1971). Zum einfluss von störtönen und störgeräuschen auf die tonhöhe von sinustönen. *Acustica*, 25, 53–61.

Thurlow, W. R. (1963). Perception of low auditory pitch: a multicue mediation theory. *Psychol. Rev.*, 70, 515–19.

Thwing, E. J. (1955). Spread of perstimulatory fatigue of a pure tone to neighboring frequencies. *J. Acoust. Soc. Am.*, 27, 741–8.

Tobias, J. V. (1963). Application of a 'relative' procedure to a problem in binaural-beat perception. *J. Acoust. Soc. Am.*, 35, 1442–7.

Tobias, J. V. (1965). Consistency of sex differences in binaural-beat perception. *Int. Audiol.*, 4, 179–82.

Tobias, J. V. (1972). Curious binaural phenomena. In *Foundations of Modern Auditory Theory*, vol. II (ed. J. V. Tobias), Academic Press, New York.

Tobias, J. V. and Schubert, E. D. (1959). Effective onset duration of auditory stimuli. *J. Acoust. Soc. Am.*, 31, 1595–605.

Tobias, J. V. and Zerlin, S. (1959). Lateralization threshold as a function of stimulus duration. *J. Acoust. Soc. Am.*, 31, 1591–4.

Tonndorf, J. (1970). Cochlear mechanics and hydro-dynamics. In *Foundations of Modern Auditory Theory* (ed. J. V. Tobias), Academic Press, New York.

References

Tumarkin, A. (1972). A biologist looks at psycho-acoustics. *J. Sound Vib.*, **21**, 115–26.

Viemeister, N. F. (1972). Intensity discrimination of pulsed sinusoids: the effects of filtered noise. *J. Accoust. Soc. Am.*, **51**, 1265–9.

Viemeister, N. F. (1974). Intensity discrimination of noise in the presence of band reject noise. *J. Acoust. Soc. Am.*, **56**, 1594–600.

Wallach, H. (1940). The role of head movements and vestibular and visual cues in sound localization. *J. Exp. Psychol.*, **27**, 339–68.

Wallach, H., Newman, E. B. and Rosenzweig, M. R. (1949). The precedence effect in sound localization. *Am. J. Psychol.*, **62**, 315–36.

Walliser, K. (1968). *Zusammenwirken von hüllkurvenperiode und tonheit bei der bildung der periodentonhöhe*, Doctoral dissertation, Technische Hochschule, München.

Walliser, K. (1969a). Zusammenhänge zwischen dem schallreiz und der periodentonhöhe. *Acustica*, **21**, 319–28.

Walliser, K. (1969b). Zur unterschiedsschwelle der periodentonhöhe. *Acustica*, **21**, 329–36.

Walliser, K. (1969c). Ueber ein funktionsschema für die bildung der periodentonhöhe aus dem schallreiz. *Kybernetik*, **6**, 65–72.

Ward, W. D. (1954). Subjective musical pitch. *J. Acoust. Soc. Am.*, **26**, 369–80.

Ward, W. D. (1963). Auditory fatigue and masking. In *Modern Developments in Audiology* (ed. J. F. Jerger), Academic Press, New York.

Ward, W. D. (1963a). Absolute pitch. Part I. *Sound*, **2**, 14–21.

Ward, W. D. (1963b). Absolute pitch. Part II. *Sound*, **2**, 33–41.

Ward, W. D. (1970). Musical perception. In *Foundations of Modern Auditory Theory*, vol. I (ed. J. V. Tobias), Academic Press, New York.

Ward, W. D., Glorig, A. and Sklar, D. L. (1958). Dependence of temporary threshold shift at 4 kc on intensity and time. *J. Acoust. Soc. Am.*, **30**, 944–54.

Warren, R. M. (1970a). Elimination of biases in loudness judgments for tones. *J. Acoust. Soc. Am.*, **48**, 1397–403.

Warren, R. M. (1970b). Perceptual restoration of missing speech sounds. *Science, N.Y.*, **167**, 392–3.

Warren, R. M. (1974). Auditory temporal discrimination by trained listeners. *Cognitive Psychol.*, **6**, 237–56.

References

Warren, R. M. (1975). Chapter in *Contemporary Issues in Experimental Phonetics* (ed. N. J. Lass), C. C. Thomas, Springfield, Ill. (in press).

Warren, R. M., Obusek, C. J., Farmer, R. M. and Warren, R. P. (1969). Auditory sequence: confusion of patterns other than speech or music. *Science, N.Y.*, **164**, 586–7.

Watson, C. S. and Gengel, R. W. (1968). Time-intensity trading relations as a function of signal frequency. *76th Meeting of the Acoustical Society of America*, paper A7.

Webster, F. A. (1951). Influence of interaural phase on masked thresholds. *J. Acoust. Soc. Am.*, **23**, 452–62.

Webster, J. C. and Muerdter, D. (1965). Pitch shifts due to low-pass and high-pass noise bands. *J. Acoust. Soc. Am.*, **37**, 382–3.

Weerts, T. C. and Thurlow, W. R. (1971). The effects of eye position and expectation on sound localization. *Percept. Psychophys.*, **9**, 35–9.

Wegel, R. L. and Lane, C. E. (1924). The auditory masking of one sound by another and its probable relation to the dynamics of the inner ear. *Phys. Rev.*, **23**, 266–85.

Weiler, M. and Friedman, L. (1973). Monaural heterophonic auditory adaptation. *J. Acoust. Soc. Am.*, **54**, Suppl., 23.

Welford, A. T. (1968). *Fundamentals of Skill*, Methuen, London.

Whitfield, I. C. (1967). *The Auditory Pathway*, Arnold, London.

Whitfield, I. C. (1970). Central nervous processing in relation to spatio-temporal discrimination of auditory patterns. In *Frequency Analysis and Periodicity Detection in Hearing* (ed. R. Plomp and G. F. Smoorenburg), Sijthoff, Leiden.

Whitfield, I. C. and Evans, E. F. (1965). Responses of auditory cortical neurones to stimuli of changing frequency. *J. Neurophysiol.*, **28**, 655–72.

Whittle, L. S., Collins, S. J. and Robinson, D. W. (1972). The audibility of low-frequency sounds. *J. Sound Vib.*, **21**, 431–48.

Whitworth, R. H. and Jeffress, L. A. (1961). Time vs intensity in the localization of tones. *J. Acoust. Soc. Am.*, **33**, 925–9.

Wiener, F. M. and Ross, D. A. (1946). The pressure distribution in the auditory canal in a progressive sound field. *J. Acoust. Soc. Am.*, **18**, 401–8.

Willey, C. F., Inglis, E. and Pearce, C. H. (1937). Reversal of auditory localization. *J. Exp. Psychol.*, **20**, 114–30.

References

Wilson, J. P. (1967). Psychoacoustics of obstacle detection using ambient or self generated noise. In *Animal Sonar Systems* (ed. R. G. Busnel), Gap, Hautes-Alpes, France.

Wilson, J. P. and Johnstone, J. R. (1972). Capacitive probe measures of basilar membrane vibrations. In *Hearing Theory*, IPO, Eindhoven.

Winckel, F. (1967). *Music, Sound and Sensation*, Dover, New York.

Wollberg, Z., and Newman, J. D. (1972). Auditory cortex of squirrel monkey: response patterns of single cells to species-specific vocalizations. *Science, N.Y.*, **175**, 212–14.

Yost, W. A., Wightman, F. L. and Green, D. M. (1971). Lateralization of filtered clicks. *J. Acoust. Soc. Am.*, **50**, 1526–31.

Young, P. T. (1928). Auditory localization with acoustical transposition of the ears. *J. Exp. Psychol.*, **11**, 399–429.

Zwicker, E. (1952). Die Grenzen der Hörbarkeit der amplitudenmodulation und der frequenzmodulation eines tones. *Acustica*, **2**, 125–33.

Zwicker, E. (1954). Die verdeckung von schmalbandgeräuschen durch sinustöne. *Acustica*, **4**, 415–20.

Zwicker, E. (1956). Die Elementaren grundlagen zur bestimmung der informationskapazität des gehörs. *Acustica*, **6**, 365–81.

Zwicker, E. (1958). Ueber psychologische und methodische grundlagen der lautheit. *Acustica*, **8** (Beih. 1), 237–58.

Zwicker, E. (1965a). Temporal effects in simultaneous masking by white-noise bursts. *J. Acoust. Soc. Am.*, **37**, 653–63.

Zwicker, E. (1965b). Temporal effects in simultaneous masking and loudness. *J. Acoust. Soc. Am.*, **38**, 132.

Zwicker, E. (1970). Masking and psychological excitation as consequences of the ear's frequency analysis. In *Frequency Analysis and Periodicity Detection in Hearing* (ed. R. Plomp and G. F. Smoorenburg), Sijthoff, Leiden.

Zwicker, E. and Fastl, H. (1972). On the development of the critical band. *J. Acoust. Soc. Am.*, **52**, 699–702.

Zwicker, E., Flottorp, G. and Stevens, S. S. (1957). Critical bandwidth in loudness summation. *J. Acoust. Soc. Am.*, **29**, 548–57.

Zwicker, E. and Scharf, B. (1965), A model of loudness summation. *Psychol. Rev.*, **72**, 3–26.

Zwicker, E. and Schutte, H. (1973). On the time-pattern of the threshold of tone impulses masked by narrow band noise. *Acustica*, **29**, 343–7.

20-2

Zwislocki, J. J. (1965). Analysis of some auditory characteristics. In *Handbook of Mathematical Psychology*, vol. 3 (ed. R. D. Luce, R. R. Bush and E. Galanter), Wiley, New York.

Zwislocki, J. J. (1969). Temporal summation of loudness: an analysis. *J. Acoust. Soc. Am.*, **46**, 431–41.

Zwislocki, J. J. (1971). Central masking and neural activity in the cochlear nucleus. *Audiology*, **10**, 48–59.

Glossary

This glossary defines most of the technical terms which appear several times in the text but which are defined only once. Sometimes the definitions are specific to the context of the book and do not apply to everyday usage of the terms.

ABSOLUTE THRESHOLD. The minimum detectable level of a sound in the absence of any other external sounds. The manner of presentation of the sound and the method of determining detectability must be specified.

AMPLITUDE. The instantaneous amplitude of an oscillating quantity (e.g. sound pressure) is its value at any instant, while the peak amplitude is the maximum value that the quantity attains. Sometimes the word peak is omitted when the meaning is clear from the context.

AUDIOGRAM. A graph showing absolute threshold for pure tones as a function of frequency. It is often plotted as hearing loss (deviation from the average threshold) in dB as a function of frequency.

AURAL HARMONIC. A harmonic generated in the auditory mechanism.

BANDWIDTH. A term used to refer to a range of frequencies. The bandwidth of a band-pass filter is often defined as the difference between the two frequencies at which the response of the filter has fallen by 3 dB (i.e. to half power).

BASILAR MEMBRANE. A membrane inside the cochlea which vibrates in response to sound and whose vibrations lead to activity in the auditory pathways. See Chapter 1.

BEATS. Periodic fluctuations which are heard when sounds of slightly different frequencies are superimposed.

BEL. A unit for expressing the ratio of two powers. The number of bels is the logarithm to the base 10 of the power ratio.

BINAURAL. A situation involving listening with two ears.

BINAURAL MASKING LEVEL DIFFERENCE (BMLD or MLD). This is a measure of the improvement in detectability of a signal which can occur under binaural listening conditions. It is the difference in threshold of the signal (in dB) for the case where the signal and masker have the same phase and level relationships at the two ears and the case where the interaural phase and/or level relationships of the signal and masker are different.

CHARACTERISTIC FREQUENCY (CF). The frequency at which the threshold of a given single neurone is lowest, i.e. the frequency at which it is most sensitive.

COMBINATION TONE. A tone perceived as a component of a complex stimulus which is not present in the sensations produced by the constituent components of the complex when they are presented alone.

COMPLEX TONE. A tone composed of a number of simple tones of different frequencies.

COMPONENT. One of the simple tones composing a complex sound. Also called a frequency component.

CYCLE. That portion of a periodic function that occurs in one period.

DECIBEL. One-tenth of a bel, abbreviated dB.

DICHOTIC. A situation in which the sounds reaching the two ears are not the same.

DIFFERENCE LIMEN (DL). Also called the just noticeable difference (jnd) or the differential threshold. The smallest detectable change in a stimulus. The method of determining detectability must be specified.

DIOTIC. A situation in which the sounds reaching the two ears are the same.

DIPLACUSIS. Binaural diplacusis describes the case when a tone of fixed frequency evokes different pitches in the left and right ear.

ENVELOPE. The envelope of any function is the smooth curve joining the peaks of the function.

EQUAL-LOUDNESS CONTOURS. Curves plotted as a function of frequency showing the Sound Pressure Level required to produce a given loudness level for a typical listener.

EXCITATION PATTERN. A term used to describe the pattern of neural activity evoked by a given sound as a function of the characteristic frequency (CF) of the neurones being excited. Sometimes the term is used to describe the effective level of excitation (in dB) at each CF.

FILTER. A device which modifies the frequency spectrum of a signal, usually while it is in electrical form.

FORMANT. A peak in the spectral envelope of a sound. The term is used particularly in describing speech sounds.

FREE FIELD. A field or system of waves free from the effects of boundaries.

FREQUENCY. For a sine wave the frequency is the number of periods occurring in one second. The unit is cycles per second, or Hz. For a complex periodic sound the term 'repetition rate' is used to describe the number of periods per second (p.p.s.).

FUNDAMENTAL FREQUENCY. The fundamental frequency of a periodic sound is that sinusoidal component of the sound that has the same period as the periodic sound.

HARMONIC. A harmonic is a component of a complex tone whose frequency is an integral multiple of the fundamental frequency of the complex. Hz. See Frequency.

INTENSITY. Intensity is the sound power transmitted through a given area in a sound field. Units such as watts per square centimetre are used. The term is also used as a generic name for any quantity relating to amount of sound, such as amplitude, level, pressure, power, etc.

LEVEL. The level of a sound is specified in dB in relation to some reference level. See Sensation Level and Sound Pressure Level.

LINEAR. A linear system is a system which satisfies the conditions of superposition and homogeneity. See Section 1.2.

LOUDNESS. This is the intensive attribute of an auditory sensation, in terms of which sounds may be ordered on a scale extending from quiet to loud.

LOUDNESS LEVEL. The Loudness Level, in phons, of a sound is the Sound Pressure Level in dB of a pure tone of frequency 1 kHz which is judged by the listener to be equivalent in loudness.

MASKED AUDIOGRAM. This is a graph of the amount of masking (in dB) produced by a given sound as a function of the frequency of the masked sound.

MASKING. Masking is the amount (or the process) by which the threshold of audibility for one sound is raised by the presence of another (masking) sound.

MASKING LEVEL DIFFERENCE (MLD). See Binaural Masking Level Difference.

MODULATION. Modulation refers to a periodic change in a particular dimension of a stimulus. Thus a sinusoid may be modulated in frequency or in amplitude.

MONAURAL. The situation in which sounds are presented to one ear only.

NOISE. Noise in general refers to any unwanted sound. White noise is a sound whose energy per unit bandwidth is constant, on average, over the range of audible frequencies. It usually has a normal (Gaussian) distribution of instantaneous amplitudes.

OCTAVE. An octave is the interval between two tones when their frequencies are in the ratio 2:1.

PARTIAL. A partial is any sinusoidal frequency component in a complex tone.

PERIOD. The period of a periodic function is the smallest time interval over which the function repeats itself.

PERIODIC SOUND. A periodic sound is one whose waveform repeats itself regularly as a function of time.

PHASE. The phase of a periodic waveform is the fractional part of a period through which the waveform has advanced, measured from some arbitrary point in time.

PHASE-LOCKING. This is the tendency for nerve firings to occur at a particular phase of the stimulating waveform.

PHON. The unit of Loudness Level.

PITCH. Pitch is that attribute of auditory sensation in terms of which sounds may be ordered on a musical scale.

PURE TONE. A sound wave whose instantaneous pressure variation as function of time is a sinusoidal function. Also called a simple tone.

RECRUITMENT. This refers to a more rapid than usual growth of loudness with increase in stimulus level, which occurs in certain types of hearing disorder.

SENSATION LEVEL. This is the level of a sound in decibels relative to the threshold level for that sound for the individual listener.

SIMPLE TONE. See Pure Tone.

SINE WAVE, SINUSOIDAL VIBRATION. A waveform whose pressure variation as a function of time is a sine function. This is the function relating the sine of an angle to the size of the angle.

SOUND PRESSURE LEVEL. This is the level of a sound in decibels relative to an internationally defined reference level. The latter corresponds to an intensity of 10^{-16} W/cm^2, which is equivalent to a sound pressure of 0.0002 dyn/cm^2 or 2×10^{-5} N/m^2.

SPECTRUM. The spectrum of a sound wave is the distribution in frequency of the magnitudes (and sometimes the phases) of the components of the wave. It can be represented by plotting power, or amplitude, or level as a function of frequency.

SPIKE. A single nerve impulse or action potential.

TIMBRE. Timbre is that attribute of auditory sensation in terms of which a listener can judge that two sounds similarly presented and having the same loudness and pitch are dissimilar. Put more simply, it relates to the quality of a sound.

TONE. A tone is a sound wave capable of exciting an auditory sensation having pitch.

TUNING CURVE. For a single nerve fibre this is a graph of the lowest sound level at which the fibre will respond, plotted as a function of frequency. Also called a frequency-threshold curve (FTC).

WAVEFORM. Waveform is a term used to describe the form or shape of a wave. It may be represented graphically by plotting instantaneous amplitude, pressure or intensity as a function of time.

Bibliography

In the past few years several very good, but fairly advanced, books on hearing have been published. Most of these have been written with the specialist in mind, and most contain chapters by several different authors, each an expert in his field. The two books which are of most general interest are *Foundations of Modern Auditory Theory*, volumes I and II, edited by J. V. Tobias (Academic Press, New York and London, 1970 and 1972). These books together cover a broad range of topics in auditory perception, and they provide an excellent review of past experiments and present knowledge (up to about 1970). Two other important and interesting books are *Frequency Analysis and Periodicity Detection in Hearing*, edited by R. Plomp and G. F. Smoorenburg (Sijthoff, Leiden, 1970) and *Basic Mechanisms in Hearing*, edited by A. R. Moller (Academic Press, New York and London, 1973). In the latter the emphasis is on anatomy and physiology rather than psychoacoustics. Both of these books are the proceedings of symposiums, and both benefit from the interesting and often illuminating discussions which follow each chapter.

Physiology of the Auditory System, edited by M. B. Sachs (National Educational Consultants, Baltimore, 1971), contains several useful papers and discussion sections, covering the physiology of the auditory system from the cochlea up to the auditory cortex, while *The Auditory Periphery*, by P. Dallos (Academic Press, New York and London, 1973), provides a very comprehensive review of the biophysics and physiology of the peripheral auditory system. *Facts and Models in Hearing*, edited by E. Zwicker and E. Terhardt (Springer-Verlag, Berlin, 1974), is the proceedings of a symposium on psychophysical models and physiological facts in hearing, and gives a good indication of recent trends in auditory research. The forthcoming book by R. Plomp, *Aspects of Tone Sensation—A Psychophysical Study* (Academic Press, London, to be published), promises to be rewarding reading, since Plomp's studies have been characterised by deep thought and great care.

There are several books which are somewhat dated but which still contain much useful information. These include *Hearing*, by S. S. Stevens and H. Davis (Wiley, New York, 1938); *The Measurement of Hearing*, by I. J. Hirsh (McGraw-Hill, New York, 1952); *Speech and Hearing in Communication*, by H. Fletcher (van Nostrand, New York, 1953); *Theory of Hearing*, by E. G. Wever (Wiley, New York, 1949); *Experiments in Hearing*, by G. von Békésy (McGraw-Hill, New York, 1960); and *Signal Detection Theory and Psychophysics*, by D. M. Green and J. A. Swets (Wiley, New York, 1966; revised edition by Kreiger, New York, 1974). The chapter by J. C. R. Licklider ('Basic correlates of the auditory stimulus') which appears in *Handbook of Experimental Psychology*, edited by S. S. Stevens (Wiley, New York), is also well worth reading.

Finally, the reader who wishes to get to the frontiers of knowledge will have to consult scientific journals! There are several important journals dealing with auditory research, but the most important is probably *The Journal of the Acoustical Society of America*, which is published monthly. Other important journals are *Acustica*, *Perception and Psychophysics*, *The Journal of Neurophysiology*, *Audiology* and the *Journal of Auditory Research*.

Index

Index